Energetic BODYWORK

Energetic BODYWORK

PRACTICAL TECHNIQUES

Rita J. McNamara

MOTILAL BANARSIDASS PUBLISHERS
PRIVATE LIMITED • DELHI

First Indian Edition: Delhi, 2002
First Published by Samuel Weiser, USA, 1998

ISBN: 81-208-1832-6

Also available at:
MOTILAL BANARSIDASS
41 U.A. Bungalow Road, Jawahar Nagar, Delhi 110 007
8 Mahalaxmi Chamber, 22 Bhulabhai Desai Road, Mumbai 400 026
236, 9th Main III Block, Jayanagar, Bangalore 560 011
120 Royapettah High Road, Mylapore, Chennai 600 004
Sanas Plaza, 1302 Baji Rao Road, Pune 411 002
8 Camac Street, Kolkata 700 017
Ashok Rajpath, Patna 800 004
Chowk, Varanasi 221 001

Printed in India
BY JAINENDRA PRAKASH JAIN AT SHRI JAINENDRA PRESS,
A-45 NARAINA, PHASE-I, NEW DELHI 110 028
AND PUBLISHED BY NARENDRA PRAKASH JAIN FOR
MOTILAL BANARSIDASS PUBLISHERS PRIVATE LIMITED,
BUNGALOW ROAD, DELHI 110 007

For
Christine, Frank, Jonathan and Michael

When we look at a tree, we see its form: the manifestation of its innate image and the result of the conditions that have governed its manifestation. Certain trees have living shapes that seem to correspond to their essential form. There are others whose bizarre contortions speak so vividly of the many storms they have endured, that it is evident that their original innate image has almost entirely disappeared or appears only as a negation of it. And yet, are not these very trees the most convincing witnesses to what happens in daily life? And does not the very manner in which they deviate from their own innate image actually reveal it?

In the same way, each individual's worldly form discloses this double origin. Unlike plants or animals, we are responsible for the extent to which our innate image is enabled to reveal itself and develop, no matter what the adverse conditions.

—from *The Way of Transformation: Daily Life as Spiritual Exercise*
by Karlfried, Graf von Durckheim
Unwin Hyman Ltd. London

CONTENTS

INTRODUCTION

Living on planet Earth during the 20th century is not the easiest thing you could have chosen to do. Like me, you've probably spent more than a few anxious moments wondering if there would be time to try to make your dreams come true, afraid sometimes to believe in a future. But when I turn aside from the television and newspaper and focus on the process that is my life and the lives around me, my sense of hope and promise is rekindled. I am continually amazed by the courage of individual lives and by the pure will to survive, to develop and to understand engendered by the human spirit.

As the millennium approaches, we are witnessing a tremendous resurgence of interest in ancient forms and systems, searching for old/new ways to know ourselves. We gently brush off the artifacts and pore over the manuscripts and scrolls, hoping to find the clue, the answer, the way to step into the future with some sense of grace and purpose. It is as though, in crossing over the psychic threshold of the year 2000, we feel the need to reach back into our dimmest past and take all the grandmothers and grandfathers with us. The burgeoning "new age" has generated countless trends, philosophies, cults, foods, gimmicks, gadgets and diets. Most of it is designed to "put us in touch with ourselves." If we peek behind the ad campaign, we often glimpse familiar patterns of competition and one-upmanship. In the same sense that our Puritan forefathers looked upon poverty as a sign of God's disfavor, many are now learning to equate physical or emotional problems with a lack of grace or spiritual balance. We have forgotten that Job's trials were the means to his evolution, his dialogue with the divine. We have forgotten that the Shaman, the one called Wounded Healer, is one who has engaged in private combat with disease and psychosis and emerged victorious, reassembled, a vehicle for power.

This book is about conflicts and patterns of tension. It is about the ways in which our past can come to haunt our present and our future. It is about the daily challenge we all confront, the challenge to somehow transmute our fears, our maimed feelings, our bitter memories and our damaged dreams. It is about our struggle to become whole, clear, and free. It is not about ways to sidestep or evade the exposure and discomfort of knowing ourselves. Nor is it about ways to numbingly detach or erase what hurts and holds us. It is a book for warriors, gentle warriors perhaps, but warriors nonetheless. For I agree with Menander the Greek who said that in being human we should "never ask the gods for life set free from grief, but ask instead for courage that endureth long."

When I was a little girl, I used to have a recurring dream about an old rainmaker. The rainmaker always seemed to be called to the most desolate, barren, God-forsaken places. The sky was sunless and yellow-grey with dust. There were only a handful of people who would meet him at the train and they were too tired to look him in the eye. They seemed old and bent before their time. He'd pick up his one shabby suitcase (rainmaking isn't all that profitable, I guess) and walk off with them. There wasn't any air of excitement or expectation or anything. Nobody seemed to think he could really make it rain. But the moviehouse was closed and there wasn't much else to do so they'd collect around. As I recall, he didn't seem to have much in the way of props or tools. He just stood around, sometimes hummed, sometimes squatted and whittled awhile on a small wooden figure he'd had in his pocket. He seemed to be waiting. The people stood about, drifted off into private thoughts, some even slept. Then after awhile a drop or two of rain would fall. You could count them, they fell so spaced and slowly. Each drop made a soft, sinking "thwop" sound as it hit the thick dust. And then it would start falling faster and faster until it was an absolute downpour. At first nobody moved. Then as the rain came faster, they'd raise their faces and stretch out their hands, not quite trusting what they saw or felt. As the reality of it took hold, they'd break into whooping, jumping pandemonium. Afterwards they said, "Well, it was probably just about to rain anyway. Had nothin' really to do with the rainmaker."

If this book could be a little like the rainmaker, bringing water to the imagination, re-uniting earth and sky, known and unknown in yourself; if it can help you to remember and reclaim a lost, forgotten freedom, a sense of wholeness and integrity, then all my work becomes a living joy.

Rita J. McNamara

CHAPTER ONE

The Living Artifact

Our forms are composed mainly of bone and muscle mass. The length of the bones and the size and shape of the muscles are largely a matter of fulfilling genetic potential. Nutrition plays the major role in the material development of these tissues. Like a tree, we develop from a particular genetic code. This code is like a blueprint, a construction plan to build a Jones-type rather than a Smith-type, in the same way that a pine becomes a pine and not an elm. And like the tree, we need nutritional substance from the earth in order to construct and manifest our form. An old tree physically reflects its encounters with storms, disasters and misfortunes. We can see how it has been fed and whether it has had to twist and turn to reach the light. We too reflect, through the silent language of posture and patterns of muscular tension, not only our genetic and nutritional status, but also how we survived and adapted to the psychological and emotional climate surrounding our development.[1]

---

[1]See Ida Rolf, *Rolfing: The Integration of Human Structures* (New York: Harper & Row, 1978); and Moshe Feldenkrais, *Awareness Through Movement* (New York: Harper & Row, 1972).

The tissues of the body become a subtle living memory of our experiences and the attitudes, beliefs and defense mechanisms we develop to survive. We are living, breathing artifacts of our own interactions with life.

We are all familiar with the ways in which the human form can be shaped and molded by repetitive movement or posture. A freight handler's upper body muscles develop differently from those of an office worker. But how is it that muscular development and body alignment can also be affected by attitude and emotion? The answer to this question is: electricity.[2]

Although bones and joints provide leverage and form the body framework, they are not capable alone of moving the body. Movement results from the contraction and relaxation of the muscle tissues attached to bones. Muscle fibers contract (shorten) or relax (lengthen) as a result of electrical charges and changes in the ionic environment of the tissues. The human body is a natural battery, generating electrical energy within a fluid ion environment. The human electromagnetic field is guided by polarity laws similar to those of classic magnetic fields. By means of the autonomic nervous system, emotional response stimulates the release of microchemicals from the endocrine glands into the bloodstream and tissues. These microchemicals alter the ionic conductivity of body tissues.[3] Emotion therefore effects the body's electrical polarity by indirectly altering the ionic environment of the cells and tissues. To understand the ways in which emotion affects specific

---

[2]See Randolph Stone, *Polarity Therapy, Wireless Anatomy of Man* (Sebastopol, CA: CRCS, 1986) and *Energy: The Vital Principle in the Healing Arts* (Sebastopol, CA: CRCS, 1974).

[3]See Kenneth Pelletier, *Mind as Healer, Mind as Slayer* (New York: Dell, 1977).

muscles and tissues, we need to understand the Oriental system of electrical body circuits called meridians.

Although Chinese medicine has much in common with Ayurvedic healing and other Oriental therapies, meridian therapy using acupuncture and acupressure is uniquely Chinese. The earliest written treatise on the subject is entitled *The Yellow Emperor's Classic of Internal Medicine*. It was written in 2697 B.C. and continues to this day to be the fundamental reference work for meridian study and therapy. The text resulted from hundreds of years of observation and recording. It was observed that particular skin areas became hypersensitive when certain illnesses and organic diseases were present in the body. These observations led to the mapping of energy points and corresponding lines or meridians on the body's surface related to the condition of internal tissues and structures. We know now that the body meridians contain a colorless, free-flowing, noncellular fluid which conveys electrical energy throughout the body. Modern science has verified and mapped the meridian circuits using advanced technological methods and equipment to track them thermally, electronically and radioactively.[4] The body's electrical circuits are divided into fourteen major meridians.

The meridians, though divided in terms of the organs and tissues they supply, actually form a continuous, single, looped circuit which conveys electromagnetic energy throughout the body. This continuous energy circuit is composed of a network of interconnections called acupoints. The acupoints are electromagnetic centers, consisting of small oval cells called

[4]See John Thie, *Touch for Health* (Marina del Rey, CA: DeVorss, 1979) page 17; and William McGarey, *Acupuncture and Body Energies* (Phoenix: Gabriel Press, 1974).

Bonham Corpuscles. Acupoints function like resistors in an electrical circuit, adjusting the speed and force of energy flow along a meridian. When body polarity is disturbed, the acupoints along the circuits respond to re-adjust the energy flow. If the polarity disturbance is recurrent or chronic, the impaired meridian flow begins to affect corresponding muscles, tissues and organs. When we understand which muscles are supplied by each meridian and how emotion impacts the meridian circuits, we are on our way to understanding how emotion and psychological conflict generate muscular tension and weakness or postural misalignment. We can begin to know how our own tree—the human body—is twisted and contorted as a result of emotional and psychological stress.

The meridians are named according to the internal structures they reflex and supply. See figures 1 and 2 on pages 6–7. There are twelve organic meridians and two storage meridians. Each of the organic meridians supplies a muscle group (or group of muscles) in the body, as well as a group of internal tissues. Six of the organic meridians are called *yin meridians*. The yin circuits convey negative electromagnetic energy throughout the body and supply the yin organs: heart, lungs, liver, spleen, kidney and circulatory vessels. The remaining six organic circuits are called *yang meridians*. The yang meridians convey positive electromagnetic energy throughout the body and supply the yang organs: stomach, large and small intestine, gall bladder, urinary bladder and adrenals.

In Oriental philosophy, the concepts of yin and yang represent the manifested duality of Oneness. Every aspect of the physical universe, from the atom to cycles of light and season, are reflective of the constant shift between polar opposites. And yet the terms yin and yang are completely relative. There is no "pure" yin, no "pure" yang. Each contains the shadow or inference of the other. The longest night of the year (yin) has been celebrated since ancient times as a festival of light (yang) because from that moment onward the days would become longer. Night follows day, rest follows action, death follows birth. When something is classified as yin—whether it is a season, an organ or a plant—it means that the qualities represented or manifested are more yin than yang. Understanding the cycles and interrelationships of yin and yang can widen and deepen understanding of ourselves and our universe. Table 1 on page 8 helps to develop and delineate concepts of yin and yang. From Table 1 we see that the feeling states which are primarily "other-directed," such as anger, intolerance and jealousy, are classified as yang; while the "self-directed" emotions, such as guilt, depression and shame, are yin.

Emotion upsets the natural balance and flow of electromagnetic energy in the body by subtly altering the chemical state of body tissues and their ionic conductivity. The yin emotions cause the body tissues to be flooded with negative electromagnetic energy. The negative congestion chokes off and deprives the yang/positive circuits and the muscles and tissues supplied by them. The converse is also true: yang emotions flood body tissues with positive electromagnetic energy and deplete the yin/negative circuits and the muscles and tissues supplied by them.

Think, for instance, of what is called the "Type A" personality—striving, perfectionistic, competitive and impatient—a very "yang" profile. Medical science has determined the Type A personality to be a prime candi-

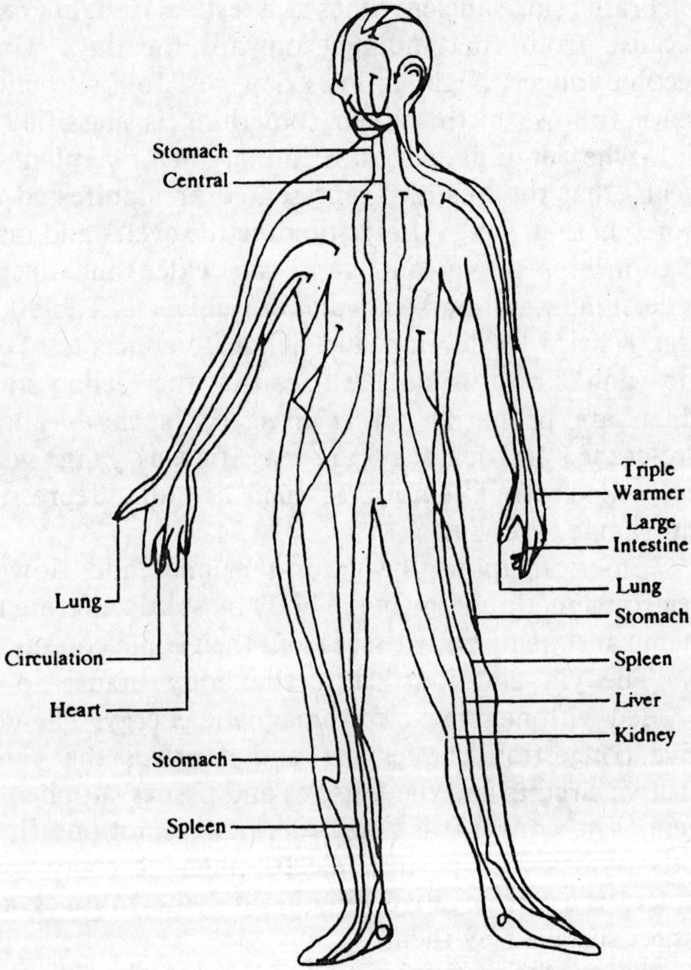

Figure 1. Front view of body meridians.

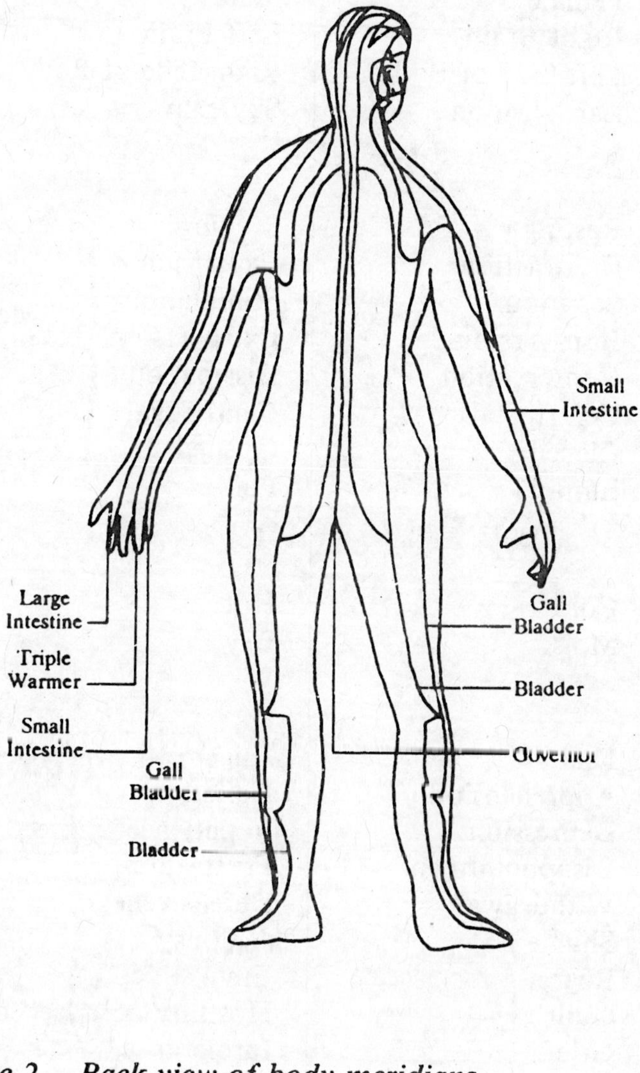

Figure 2. Back view of body meridians.

Table 1. Yin and Yang Polarities.

Yin	Yang	
Negative Polarity	Positive Polarity	
Female	Male	
Right Brain	Left Brain	
Left Side of Body	Right Side of Body	
Earth/Moon	Sky/Sun	
Resting	Moving	Moving States
Contraction	Expansion	
Sedation	Stimulation	
Introversion	Extroversion	
Conservation	Dissipation	
Centripetal	Centrifugal	
Closed	Opened	
Empty	Full	
Cold	Hot	
Moist	Dry	
Fear	Anger	
Apprehension	Agitation	Feeling States
Depression	Impatience	
Disappointment	Frustration	
Withdrawal	Defensiveness	
Shame	Jealousy	
Regret	Envy	
Guilt	Hostility	
Grief	Intolerance	

date for heart and blood vessel diseases.[5] The yang Type A conflicts and emotions weaken and deplete the yin organs, the heart and blood vessels. The meridian section of this book describes each of the organic meridians in detail and outlines, among other things, the types of emotion and conflict which weaken the meridian and the tissues it supplies. For now, it is important only to understand that the yang emotions represented by states of agitation and over-involvement overload the positive electromagnetic polarity circuits and deprive the negative channels. The yin emotions, represented by states of fear and withdrawal, overload the negative polarity body circuits and deplete the positive ones. This is basically how emotion and conflict electrochemically affect body tissues.

We know that just as calm follows the storm, no one is permanently angry or sad. Yesterday's gloominess gives way to today's lighter attitude. The emotional balance moves back and forth, yin to yang, shifting organic polarity in its wake. Since the body polarity is constantly adjusting and changing, attempting to return to balance and homeostasis, why should there be any imprinting, any "memory" left behind on muscles or tissues? Why isn't the body-mind slate wiped clean after each shift, experiencing the moment's reality, unmindful of former states?

This is a complex question. One of the answers is that, as humans, we possess the ability to reflect, to remember and to visualize. We can hold images, memories, and fantasies in our mind's eye. These are mental constructs—they do not, in fact, appear before us. But the internal body reacts to them as though we were

[5]Pelletier, *Mind as Healer, Mind as Slayer.*

experiencing them in actuality.[6] A fearful dream stimulates the autonomic nervous system as though we were experiencing the alarming scenario in the "real" world. We relive some emotions and conflicts again and again through the mechanism of memory, dream, and recollection. Another part of the answer to this question involves the body's glandular centers.

There are seven glandular centers, sometimes called chakras, within the body. The glandular centers function like transducers along the two main storage meridians. Each time there is a shift in organic polarity, there is a shift in the chakra center energies. The chakras regulate the exchange and transfer of polarity energies and record the reason for the transaction. In this way each of the chakra centers becomes an electromagnetic accumulator, or data bank, storing information about the nature and type of the organism's polarity shifts. This is why an individual receiving a polarity treatment will often experience revelatory emotional sensations, sometimes briefly reliving or re-experiencing an emotional episode from the past. By activating the centers through the electromagnetic shifts in the treatment, images and feelings are often startlingly released.

The chakra centers, as body-mind memory banks, appear at first to be a distinct physical and psychological disadvantage. Because of them, we seem to be at the mercy of both today's and yesterday's emotional expenditures. The chakra centers appear to be seven implements of torture, capable of keeping us in a state of continual electrochemical stress. Why should we be fitted with mechanisms of such doubtful merit? Perhaps

---

[6]Michael and Nancy Samuels, *Seeing with the Mind's Eye* (New York: Random House, 1975).

we need to examine our most basic and ancient understandings of ourselves as beings to determine how these centers implement our evolution.

Our oldest bio-cosmologies describe the human being as an entity resident not only on the physical, three-dimensional plane, but as a complex being composed of several bodies both phenomenal and non-phenomenal. The non-phenomenal bodies provide the vehicle for evolution and development on levels other than the purely physical. In these systems, the seven glandular centers (chakras) serve as a communicational network between the physical body and its subtler counterparts.[7]

In the Egyptian System of the Five Bodies,[8] the vehicles are described as interpenetrating and interactive. Each of the bodies has a dimension and function of its own. The goal of human evolution, as understood from this perspective, is the full development of each of the bodies while consciously, functionally, integrating all five. See figure 3 on page 12 for an illustration of the chakras and the Egyptian system of the Five Bodies.

The body we are most familiar with is the physical body of organs, blood, bone and muscle. It is the organic earth body, named in the Egyptian system, *Aufu*. It is this body which houses the seven glandular centers (chakras). The bodies communicate with each other by means of these chakra centers. The chakras, in

[7]Hiroshi Motoyama and R. Brown, *Science and Evolution of Consciousness: Chakras, Ki & Psi* (Brookline, MA: Autumn Press, 1978).
[8]For a complete exposition of the cosmology of bodies in Egyptian mythology and spiritual discipline, see Robert Masters, "The Way of the Five Bodies," *Aquarian Changes*, Vol. 5 No. 2, April, 1983. Masters has also just published a book-length treatment of this subject titled *The Goddess Sekhmet: The Way of the Five Bodies* (Warwick, NY: Amity House, 1988).

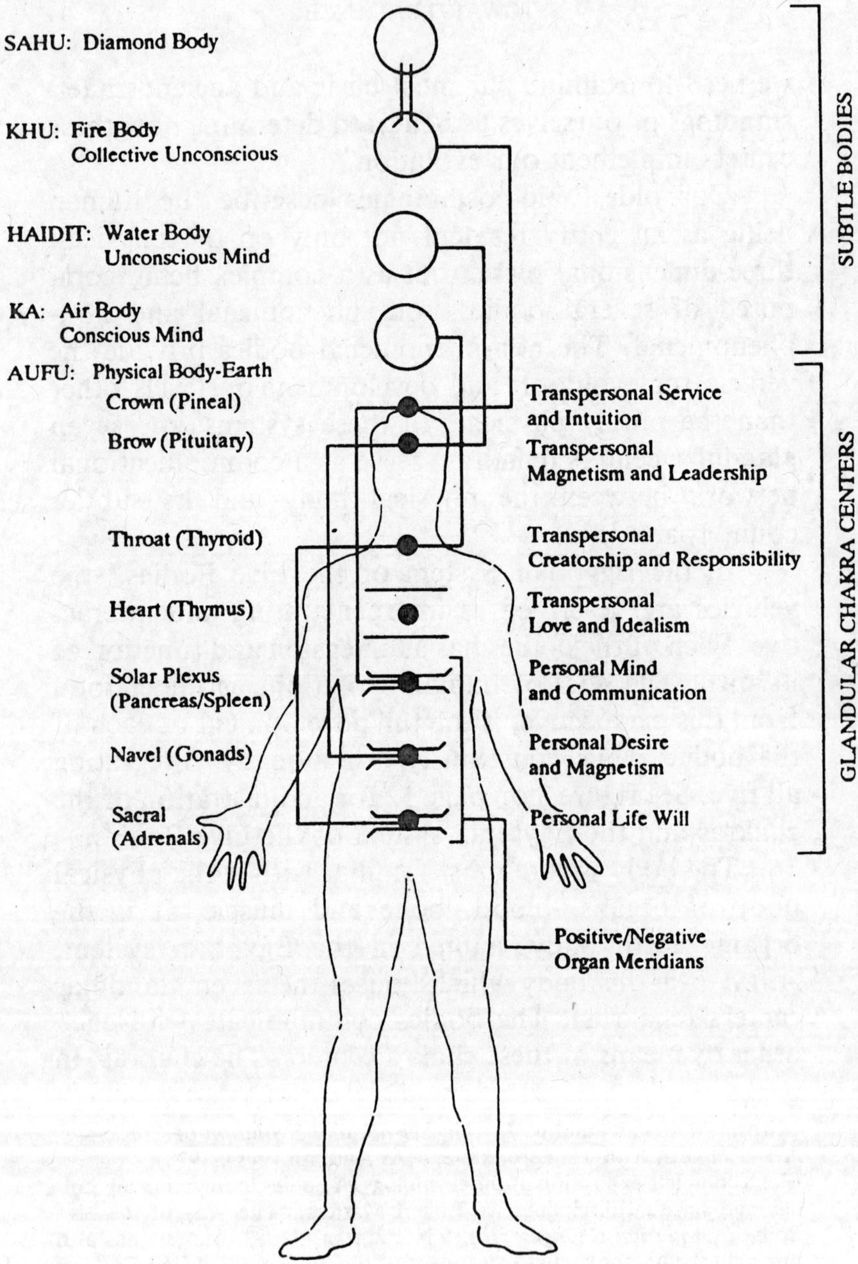

Figure 3. The chakra centers and the five subtle bodies.

turn, influence every organ and tissue of the physical body via a network of subtle energy circuits (meridians). From this perspective, it is understood that the condition of the physical body can both effect and/or result from energy states in the other bodies. It is also understood that what we do with the physical vehicle—how we feed and move it, how we care for it, the environments we expose it to, even how we dress or adorn it—can reflex the chakra glandular centers through the meridian channels and effect not only the physical body itself, but also the hidden bodies. In the Egyptian system, the true function of the physical body is to serve as an instrument of the subtle bodies (and their forces) in the three-dimensional world.

The second body described by the Egyptian system is called the *Ka*. It represents the conscious mind or intellectual body, the body of Air. Ka's world or dimension is more subtle than Aufu's. Aufu's dimension—the physical world of form—is actually shaped and held intact by the work of the Ka body. Ka's true task is to strengthen itself through concentration and self-observation in order to become a disciplined and consistent form-builder. In an undeveloped state, the Ka is a reservoir of patterned/conditioned thought and attitude which unconsciously orchestrates physical reality. The developed Ka body becomes a bridge between the dream body and the physical vehicle, making conscious the unconscious. Today there is increasing research into, and evidence of, the relationship between mind and body, between thought and form. The marketplace is jammed with information on ways to recondition the intellect and consequently affect the physical self and its environment. These range from positive thinking and psycho-cybernetics to meditation and hypnosis for the purposes of behavior modification. The reason why so many of these methods, basically sound in principle, may produce initially dramatic effects but fail in the long run, is that many conditioned thoughts and attitudes have imprinted themselves in the muscles and tissues of the body via the glandular centers and meridians. These conditionings must be cleared, not only from the intellectual body, but also from the muscles and tissues in order to stop the pattern from reinstating itself. The muscular and postural vocabulary, a potent electrochemical language, keeps "talking" to the body tissues and overrides short sessions of mental retraining or hypnosis.

The third body in the Egyptian system is called the *Haidit.* It is the body of the unconscious mind, the Water body. In some traditions it is called the double, the dream or astral body, or the shadow. The Haidit body is functional in the landscape of myth, art and dream. Through lucid dreaming, the Haidit's task is to detachedly explore the contents of the unconscious and integrate its reality with the physical reality (Aufu's level) through the medium of the conscious mind (Ka's level). In this way the physical self is empowered by the personal myth and armed with a wider range of creative expression and resolution with which to confront and resolve the conflicts of physical reality.

The Fire or "magical" body is the body of the collective consciousness. In the Egyptian system it is called *Khu*. The Khu body is functional on the archetypal level of being. It is on this level that one contacts the teacher or "master." This is why it is so often said that "when the pupil is ready, the teacher appears." The teacher is always resident within oneself and accessed through the proper alignment and function of the subtle bodies.

Alignment can only occur when particular work—physical, mental and emotional—has been done to affect the glandular chakra centers. A physical teacher may point the way to this work and even assist in the process, but only the individual can do the work and awaken to the teacher within. True psycho-physical work in healing and transformation is activated from this level of inner guidance. The hope and goal of the Khu body is to become a channel for the higher self into the physical plane.

The fifth body in the Egyptian system is called the *Sahu*. In some traditions it is called the luminous or transfigured body, or the diamond body. It is the body which links the human level with the God or Divine level of being. The work of the Sahu body is to attempt permeation of the lower bodies, through the Khu, in order to enable the highest level of work and purpose to evolve on the physical plane.

In the Egyptian system of the Five Bodies, we find a metaphor for alchemical work. The separated elements—Earth, Air, Fire and Water—symbolized by the four lower bodies, are refined and realigned into the reality of the Fifth—the indestructible Diamond Self, the Philosopher's Stone—the symbol of unity and realization.[9]

The ancient Egyptian system illuminates a great deal, not only concerning the function of the chakra centers, but also concerning our purpose as total beings and the function of health and dis-ease in our lives.

Through the lens of the Egyptian system, we see that accumulations, blockages, and imbalances at the chakra center level represent evolutionary challenges to

---

[9] A. E. Waite, *The Hermetical & Alchemical Writings of Paracelsus* (Boston: Shambhala, 1976).

resolve in order to progress toward a more perfect expression of The Work. Though chakra center imbalances may produce physical "symptoms" via the glandular and meridian networks, this is not because the body itself is "sick," but because it is being crippled in carrying out its higher function. By confronting and studying each chakra imbalance and the challenge it represents, we can learn what we have placed in the way of our greater perfection. Using this system of diagnosis, imbalance and dis-ease become motivational and directional data—and not just a set of unpleasant physical or emotional sensations! The Egyptian system teaches us that stress on any level of being (whether or not we refer to it as a "body") can create or result from stress on other levels. A human being is not compartmentalized into areas of emotional, mental, spiritual and organic function which have no relationship or communication with one another.

The vibrational therapies which specifically impact the glandular chakra centers represent the healing forms of the future as we strive to become conscious, rhythmic instruments in physical reality. They are as follows:

Polarity—Electromagnetic Pulse Balancing
Meridian Therapy
Aromatherapy
Homeopathic Remedies
Chromotherapy & Gemstone Therapy

We will discuss these therapies in more detail in the following chapters.

CHAPTER TWO

Working with the Chakras

Our evolution as integrated individuals depends on our ability to confront, resolve and adapt to life conflicts. Nearly every theory of personality development employs a stage or phase model which presents internal conflict as the primary teacher of the evolving personality. Periods of anxiety, confusion and doubt are our chances, psychologically, to "make the growth choice rather than the fear choice."[10] The chakra centers constitute both physiological mechanisms and psychological models of personality growth. Each center is a collecting point, electrochemically, for a particular area of conflict and development. The chakras function like transducers along the two main electrical circuits in the body (see figure 4 on page 18). They regulate exchanges in organic polarity and record each electromagnetic transaction. Since many of the shifts in organic polarity result indirectly from emotional response, the chakras

[10]Abraham Maslow, "Self-Actualization and Beyond" in *Challenges in Humanistic Psychology* (New York: McGraw-Hill, 1967), page 282.

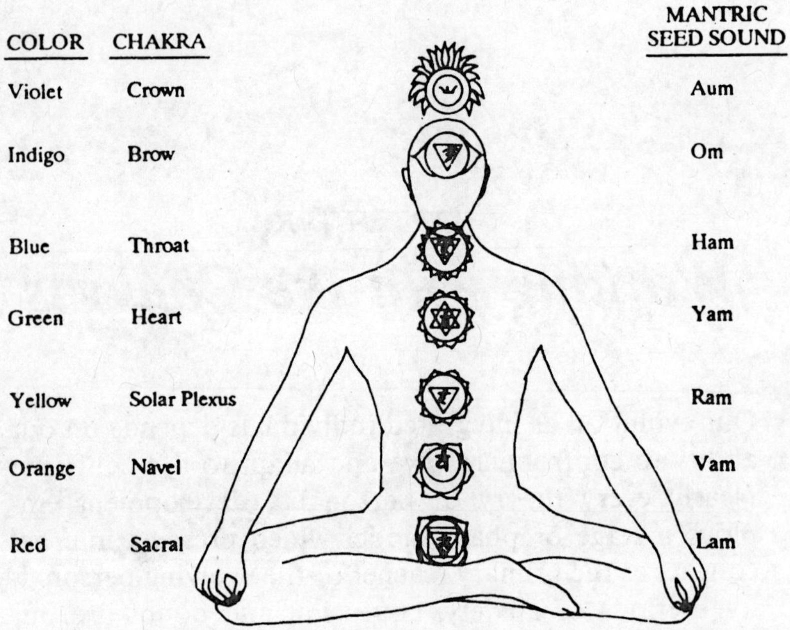

Figure 4. The chakra centers and ancient vibrational patterns (yantra) corresponding to each center.

become data banks, storing information about individual conflicts and experiential impressions.

The three lower chakras—the sacral, navel and solar plexus centers—represent the basic life centers. These are the physical/moving center (sacral), the emotional/desire center (navel) and the mental/communicating center (solar plexus). Psychologically, the lower centers represent developmental areas of personal will:

The Will-To-Be – Sacral
The Will-To-Have – Navel
The Will-To-Know – Solar Plexus

The three higher centers – the throat, brow and crown – are higher vibrational octaves of the basic life centers. The higher centers function as direct links between the physical vehicle and the subtle (or non-physical) bodies. As such they might be termed the Transpersonal Centers. The higher centers can consistently function only after the electromagnetic energies of the lower centers have been recycled and redirected onto the higher vibrational level. Most of us spend the bulk of our energies struggling with the conflicts and impressions attached to the lower centers. In this way we are held prisoner of experience, conflict, attitude and belief, and the higher centers are denied the force necessary to their own development and function. Our links with the non-physical vehicles are therefore tentative and erratic, and higher level growth is retarded. Only consistent work on the lower centers can liberate the energy necessary to activate the higher centers and consciously, resonantly forge the bonds between the subtle bodies and the physical vehicle. The higher centers represent developmental areas of transpersonal will:

The Will-To-Create – Throat
The Will-To-Leadership – Brow
The Will-To-Service – Crown

Figure 3 on page 12 schematically represents the relationship between the higher and lower centers. It also shows the relationship between the higher centers and the non-physical bodies.

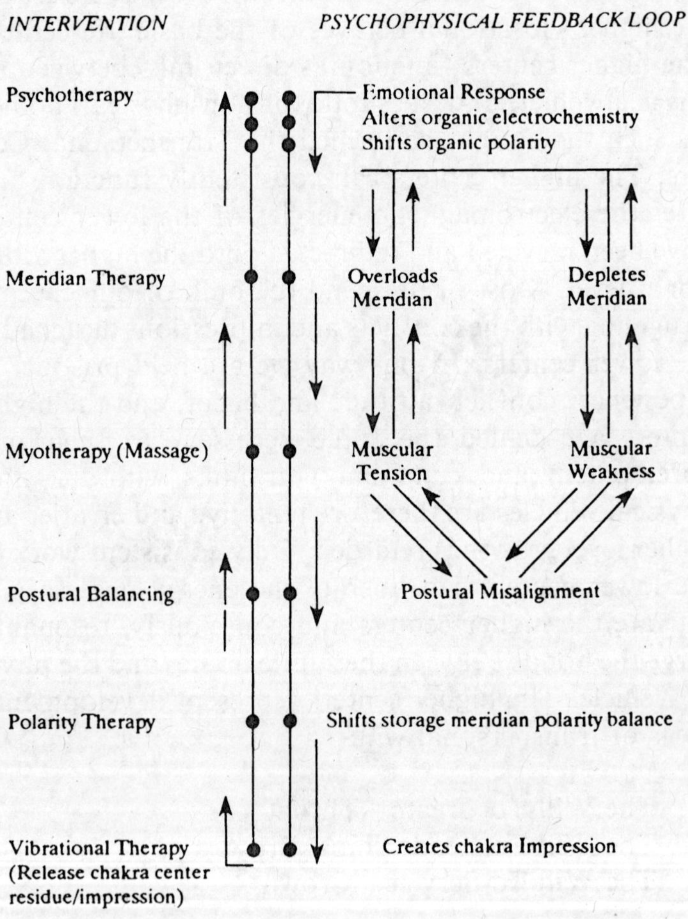

Figure 5. Therapeutic intervention interrupts and reprograms the psychophysical patterning cycle.

The heart center functions as an initiatic center. It transforms energies from the personal to the transpersonal level. Psychologically, the heart center represents the Will-To-Love, the urge for expansion of being and the connection with higher orders of development.

The twelve organic meridians network to and from the main storage circuits and chakra centers. Because the meridians network to *and from* the centers, body muscles and tissues can become affected by impressions and conflict patterns stored at the chakra level. Working to release residues at the chakra level alters the electrical energies conveyed by the meridian circuits, and reflexly affects the muscles and tissues supplied by them. At the same time, releasing tensions held in the posture and muscles alters the meridian energies and impacts the chakra centers. Integrated therapy requires intervention along the entire psycho-physical feedback loop.[11] To significantly change patterns of stress, we need to strive for balance on both the organic and psychological level. Figure 5 provides a graphic representation of a psychophysical feedback loop, a complex pattern of cause and effect, and the types of therapeutic interventions which can interrupt and alter the psychophysical pattern.

---

[11]See Gregory Bateson, "Cybernetic Explanation" in *Steps to an Ecology of Mind* (New York: Ballantine, 1972) pages 403–404, specifically his comments on the concept of feedback: "When the phenomena of the universe are seen as linked together by cause and effect and energy transfer, the resulting picture is of complexly branching and interconnecting chains of causation . . . events at any position in the circuit may be expected to have effect at all positions on the circuit at later times." A psycho-physical feedback circuit involves just such a complex causation chain involving emotions, autonomic nervous system response, altered electrochemistry, and so on.

TESTING THE CHAKRAS

Assessing the chakra centers to detect electrochemical accumulations is a simple matter of radiesthesia.[12] The individual to be assessed is positioned supine (lying on the back) with the head in a northerly or easterly direction. The assessor-therapist suspends a pendulum directly over each of the chakra centers along the storage meridian (see figure 6). The energy vortex at each center should be turning in a clockwise direction. The force and direction of the pendulum movement will indicate the energy state at the chakra level.[13] If the pendulum moves in any direction other than clockwise while suspended over a particular center, it indicates an imbalance or electrochemical accumulation at that center.

Chakra center disturbances may be either acute or chronic in nature. An acute imbalance represents a temporary state or phase of electrochemical disequilibrium. The acute disturbance is usually the result of short term conflicts and current life challenges. An acute imbalance has not produced postural and muscular patterns because it has not been ingrained in the psychophysical feedback loop long enough to do so.

A chronic imbalance, on the other hand, represents a state of recurring electrochemical disequilibrium. This type of imbalance is repetitive, a pattern of longer duration and one that has begun to produce degenerative

---

[12]Radiesthesia is the term used to indicate dowsing an area with a pendulum to detect fluctuations in an electromagnetic field.

[13]For descriptions of radiesthesia and pendulum movements in assessing vortex energies, see Tom Graves, *The Diviner's Handbook* (Rochester, VT: Inner Traditions, 1977), and H. Tomlinson, *The Divination of Disease: A Study of Radiesthesia*,now out of print but worth reading if you can find a copy.

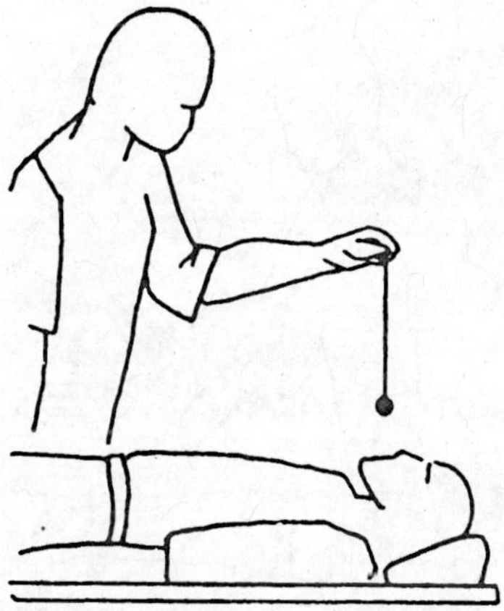

Figure 6. Testing the chakra centers.

effects in reflexed muscles and tissues. The chronic imbalance is always accompanied by corresponding postural and muscular tension. It signifies a fixed psychological pattern which has clearly begun to imprint on body tissues. This type of pattern has been ingrained in the psychophysical feedback loop long enough to electrochemically generate muscular "pictures."

Each chakra center imbalance or disturbance should be traced through the meridians networking to/from the disturbed center. Examining the muscles supplied by the meridians will clearly identify postural imbalances if they exist, and separate the acute from the chronic imbalance.

Acute chakra imbalances can often be completely cleared and released by winding the disturbed center. Winding the center retrains the energy at the chakra vortex. To wind the chakra vortex, the assessor-therapist makes several clockwise circular passes over

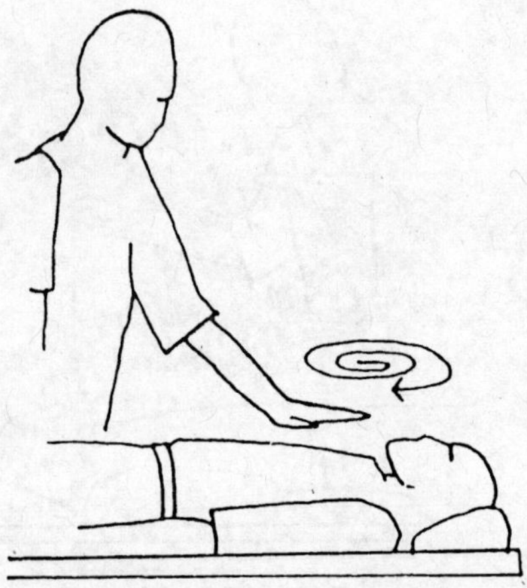

Figure 7. Winding.

the chakra center (see figure 7). An acute imbalance can be temporarily realigned in this manner.

Chronic imbalances require more extensive intervention and retraining. The first step in effectively working with chronic chakra center accumulations is to identify which meridian is habitually being affected by the imbalance. This is done through the careful assessment of the muscles supplied/reflexed by the center's meridians. For example, suppose the chakra assessment uncovers an imbalance at the solar plexus center. We know immediately that the psychological conflict underlying the disturbance involves some aspect of the individual's integration of mental and communicational energies, because the solar plexus center is the accumulator for this type of developmental conflict. The meridians networking to/from the solar plexus center are the spleen, stomach, kidney, and urinary bladder. We check the postural and muscular "pictures" that result from chronic depletion and weakening of these meridians. In doing so, we discover that the client holds one shoulder higher than the other—a muscular picture associated with depletion of the spleen meridian. The psychosocial conflict that weakens the spleen meridian is one of mental superiority, the need to intellectually dominate and "convert" others. It is a profile of mental rigidity which, in the extreme, can manifest as narrow-mindedness, bias and prejudice. By locating the meridian weakness and its accompanying postural picture, we have clearly identified the conflict which is reinstating imbalance. This opens up a range of retraining options:

1) psychological counseling appropriate to the identified conflict;

2) homeopathic treatment to facilitate release of related psycho-social stresses;

3) myotherapy to retrain affected muscles and realign posture;

4) meridian and polarity therapy to readjust imbalanced organic electrical circuits;

5) vibrational therapy to assist in releasing chakra center residues and accumulations.

PULSE POINT BALANCING

Each chakra is accompanied by a set of pulses that function like resistors to readjust the chakra energies. In using the pulse points, the healer creates a temporary circuit with his or her hands and body in order to balance and realign chakra energies. The healer places hands or fingertips lightly on the pulse points, waiting to sense a slight rhythmic unison with one another. The healer may also sense a temperature difference between the two pulse locations. The healer holds the pulses lightly until they are synchronized, pulsing in unison, and even in temperature. A pulse balancing at each location may require thirty seconds to two minutes or more.

The polarity pulse point sequence, a series of movements and balancings, realigns each chakra and can be used as a gentle, relaxing form of bodywork.

WORKING WITH THE CHAKRA TABLES

In the following pages, we will examine each of the chakras in more detail from physical, psychological and therapeutic viewpoints. To make study of each chakra as easy as possible, and to provide therapists with a clear reference guide, the chakra section is set out in table format. Then each chakra table provides several categories and areas of information, including:

Location: The location of the chakra center and radiesthesia testing position.

Developmental challenge: A description of the developmental challenge that each chakra center represents. The needs, urges and conflicts which arise from this area of growth and which may cause electrochemical accumulation at the chakra center.

Physical states: A description of the physical states that may accompany or engender center disturbance.

Vitamin/mineral: Any vitamin/mineral deficiency that may result from or cause center imbalance.

Polarity therapy treatment points: Each chakra is accompanied by a set of pulse points that function like resistors to readjust the chakra energies and main storage meridian balance. In using the pulse points, healers create a temporary circuit with their own hands/body to realign the chakra energies. A description of point location and instructions for balancing are included in each table under each chakra section.

Meridians: This section in the tables lists the four meridians which network to/from the center, linking physical tissues with the chakra center. When a chakra center imbalance is detected, each of its four meridians, and the meridian muscles, must be examined to determine whether or not the chakra disturbance has begun to electrochemically imprint on the body tissues and create a psychophysical feedback loop. Isolating the affected meridian clearly identifies the psycho-social conflict underlying the disturbance and locates the body circuit and muscular tissues which need readjustment. Instructions for locating each meridian, detecting imbalances, and readjusting meridian energies is found in chapter 3, "Working with Meridians." Myotherapy techniques for releasing muscular tension and strengthening weakened muscles is also found in this section. Bracketed page numbers in the chakra tables refer you to specific meridians which network to and from the chakra center.

Aromatherapy: Aromatherapy is a vibrational form of treatment which stimulates the release of residues, impressions, and blockages held at the center level. Each chakra center has a specific anointing point which reflexes it. Several essential oils will affect each center. To use aromatherapy, *one* essential oil is selected and applied to the chakra anointing point. Refer also to chapter 4, "Vibrational Therapies."

Homeopathic remedies: Treatment with homeopathic remedies assists in releasing emotional and psychological stresses. Several remedies are listed for each chakra center. These selected remedies have been found to be consistently useful in treatment of the type of stresses associated with various chakra developmental areas. Profiles for the remedies, and instructions for preparing and using them, will be found in chapter 4, "Vibrational Therapies."

Color & Gemstone: Color and gemstone therapy is a vibrational form of treatment which stimulates the release of residues, impressions, and blockages held at the chakra center level. Each chakra center has a specific color and gemstone which stimulates and reflexes it. Treatment forms and procedures for using color and gemstones to balance the chakra energies are detailed in chapter 4.

SACRAL CHAKRA CENTER

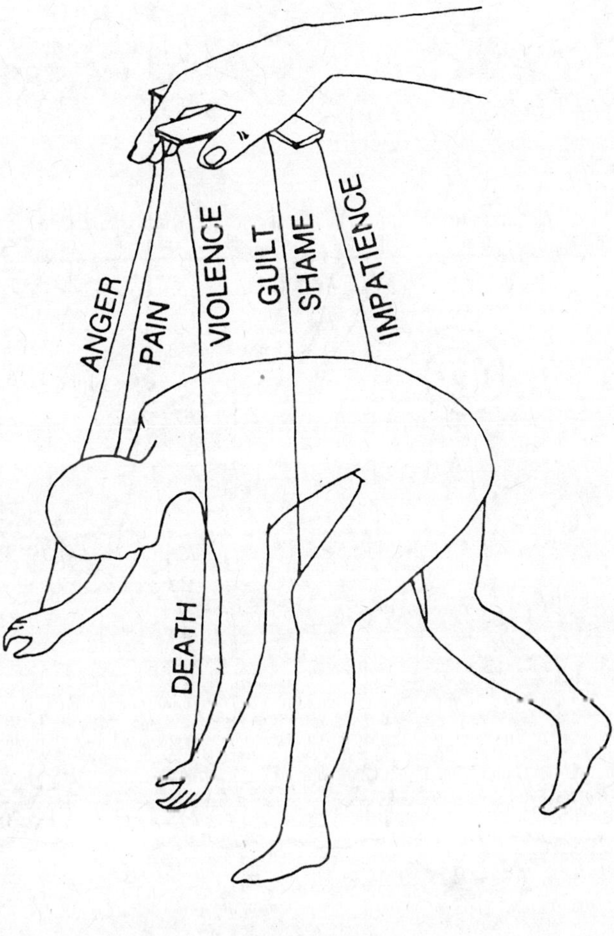

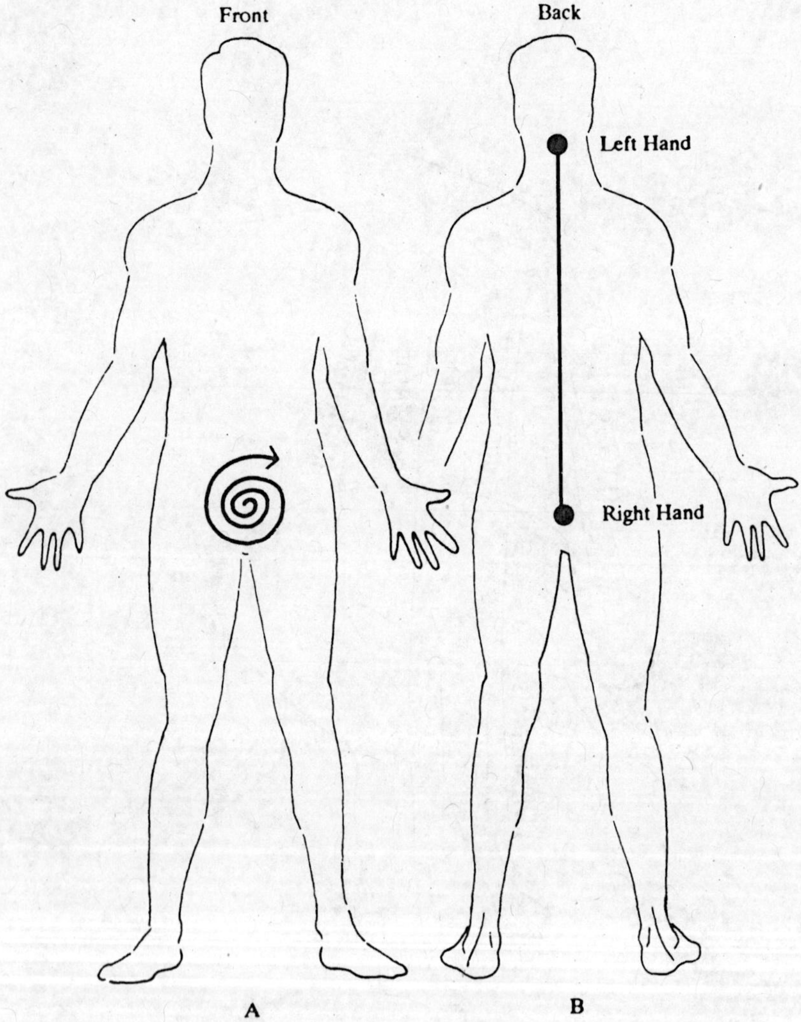

Figure 8. The root chakra. (A) shows the location of the chakra and (B) shows the balance points.

Location

The sacral chakra center is located at the base of the spine in the pelvic basin. To assess sacral center energies, position the person supine (lying on the back) and suspend the pendulum directly over the pelvic area (see figure 8A, front view). To realign sacral center energies, position the person prone (lying on the stomach) and use the pulse points described under "Polarity Therapy Treatment Points" and see figure 8B (back view).

Developmental Challenge: The Will to Be

The sacral chakra is the organic and esoteric center corresponding with the adrenal glands. It is the psychological center for the evolution of personal will to identity and autonomy and the urge for action and survival. Included in this developmental area are the urge for personal significance, individuality and self-expression, and the need for safety, self-esteem, achievement and recognition. The sacral center is the electrochemical accumulator for impressions, memories, conflicts, attitudes and beliefs engendered in our efforts to achieve personal autonomy and identity. Early negative patterning concerning

- the safety of our environment and guardians
- the appropriateness and effectiveness of our actions and expressions
- the expectations of our gender or cultural role

can chronically imprint the sacral center and create a negative psychophysical feedback loop.

The sacral center can become temporarily (acutely) disturbed following shock, trauma, accident, fright, injury, or exposure to threat or danger. The sacral center will also be disturbed during phases of sexual transition, such as puberty, pregnancy, menopause, mid-life crisis, reproductive system surgery or injury, or during periods of any significant change in sexual activity or behavior.

Psychological States

Psychological states associated with sacral imbalance include gender or cultural role confusion, identity crisis, fear, regret, shame, shyness, timidity, victimization, martyrdom, inferiority, anger, aggression, impatience, intolerance, self-absorption, pride, self-pressuring, competitiveness.

Physical States

Those associated with sacral imbalance include anaemia, iron deficiency, poor or spasmodic circulation, low blood pressure, poor muscle tone, fatigue, adrenal insufficiency.

Polarity Therapy Treatment Points

To balance, position the recipient prone (lying on the stomach). Healer places his or her left hand at the base of the skull, and right hand at the end of the spine (see figure 8B). The left hand is held steady, while the right hand begins a gentle, rocking motion of the lower back and pelvis. The body may resist rocking at first, but the motion should be maintained until some freedom of movement is established in the lower back. Then, both hands are held quietly and steadily, sensing the pulse in each location. Hands are held in place until an even temperature is sensed in both locations and both locations are pulsing in an even, synchronized way.

Meridians

Heart (page 87), circulation (page 89), triple warmer (page 91), small intestine (page 93).

Aromatherapy

Clove oil (*Caryophyllus*), Basil oil (*Ocymum basilicum*), Neroli oil (*Citris vulgaris*). The anointing point is the base of the brain, just above hairline.

Homeopathic Remedies

Mullein, Wild Rose, Hellebore, Crabapple, Pine, Comfrey, Walnut, Wild Oat, Hyssop, Nightshade, Poison Ivy, Leopard's-bane, Monkshood.

Correspondences

Color: red, *Planet*: Sun/Mars, *Vitamin/mineral*: E and iron, *Gland*: adrenal, *Gemstone*: carnelian, *Musical tone*: C.

NAVEL CHAKRA CENTER

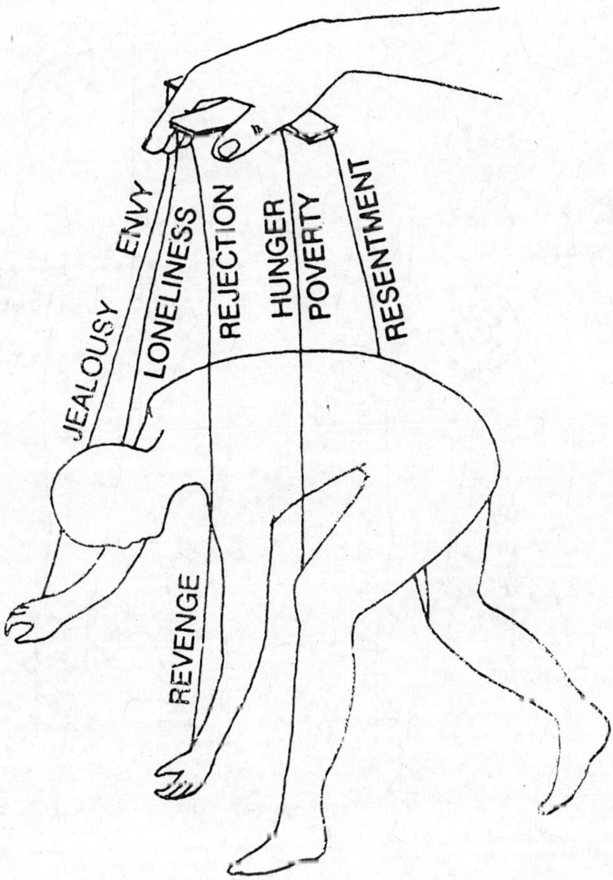

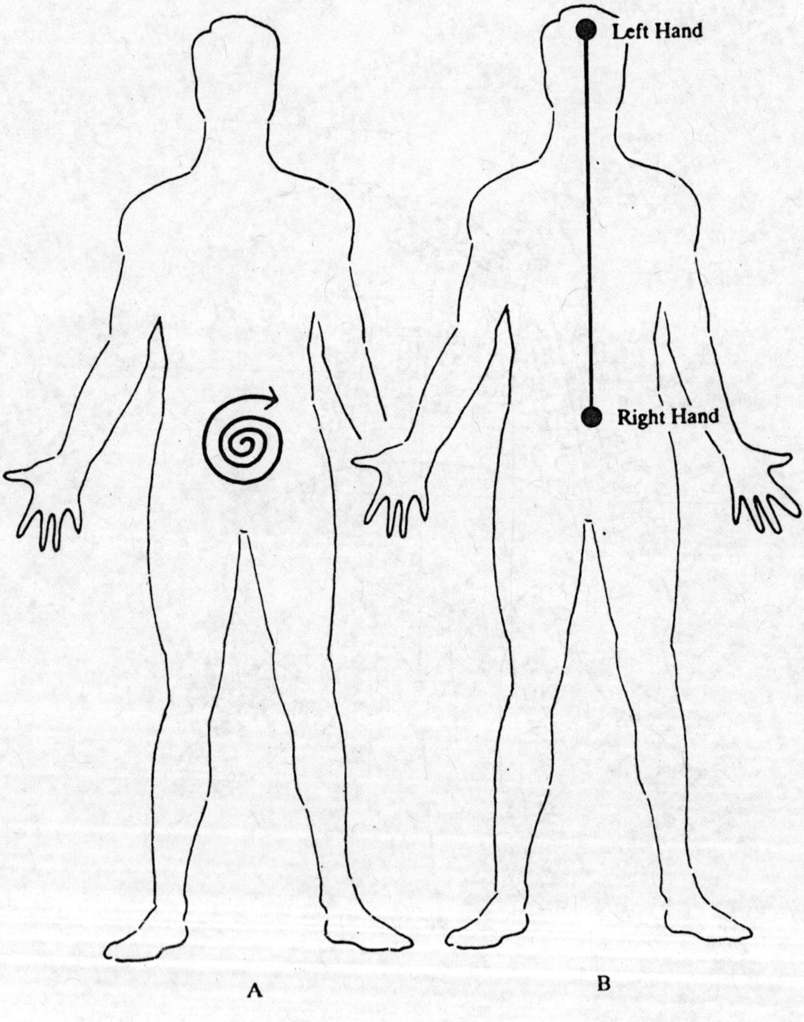

Figure 9. The navel chakra. (A) shows the chakra location; (B) shows the balancing points.

Location

The navel center is located at the navel area, commonly called the "belly button." To assess navel center energies, position the person supine (lying on the back) and suspend the pendulum directly over the navel area (see figure 9A, front view). Balance treatment points are located on the front of the body. To realign navel center energies, work on the front of the body and use the pulse points described under "Polarity Therapy Treatment Points" on page 38.

Developmental Challenge: The Will to Have

The navel chakra is the organic and esoteric center corresponding with the gonads. It is the psychological center for the evolution of the personal desire and emotion force, the will to have and love, and the urge for security and belonging. Included in this developmental area are the urge for stability (both materially and emotionally) and the need for affection and security. The navel center is the electrochemical accumulator for impressions, memories, conflicts, attitudes and beliefs engendered in our efforts to establish a viable support system. Early negative patterning concerning

- the security/stability of the emotional and material support system;
- our attractiveness, desirability, and right to be loved;
- experiences with lack or abundance (poverty, hunger, etc.)

chronically imprint the navel center and create a negative psychophysical feedback loop. The navel center may become temporarily (acutely) disturbed during periods of relationship stress, divorce, separation, loss and abandonment, and also as a result of theft, loss or damage to the material support system (possessions, job, income). Episodes that damage self-image, or make us feel unattractive or self-conscious, will also disturb the navel center.

Psychological States

Those associated with disturbance of the navel center are possessiveness, greed, hoarding, fears of loss, hunger, poverty, abandonment, relationship confusion or hostility, defensiveness, jealousy, envy, loneliness, hatred, resentment, feelings of neglect or being unappreciated, self-consciousness, fear of aging.

Physical States

Physical states associated with imbalance of the navel center include respiratory and bronchial disorders, muscular spasms, cramping and crippling, menstrual disorders and hormonal imbalances, exposure to environmental poisons, toxins and pollutants.

Polarity Therapy Treatment Points

To balance, position the recipient supine (on the back). Healer places his or her left hand on the forehead and right hand over the navel, as shown in figure 9B. The left hand is held steady, while the right hand begins a gentle rocking of the abdomen. The body may resist rocking at first, but the rocking motion should be maintained until some freedom of movement is established in the abdominal area. Then, both hands are held steadily and quietly in place until an even temperature is sensed in both locations and the pulses in both locations are beating in unison.

Meridians

Lung (page 95), liver (page 97), gall bladder (page 99), and large intestine (page 101).

Aromatherapy

Chamomile oil (*Anthemis nobilis*), Wintergreen oil (*Gaultheria procumbens*). Anointing points are brow and middle of the forehead.

Homeopathic Remedies

Holly, Mallow, St. Johnswort, Hawthorn, Walnut, Willow, Hyssop, Wild Rose, Hellebore, Ignatius, Stavesacre, Jasmine, Chamomile.

Correspondences

Color: orange, *Planet*: Moon/Venus, *Vitamin/Mineral*: B complex and calcium, *Gland*: gonads, *Gemstone*: amber, *Musical tone*: D.

SOLAR PLEXUS CHAKRA CENTER

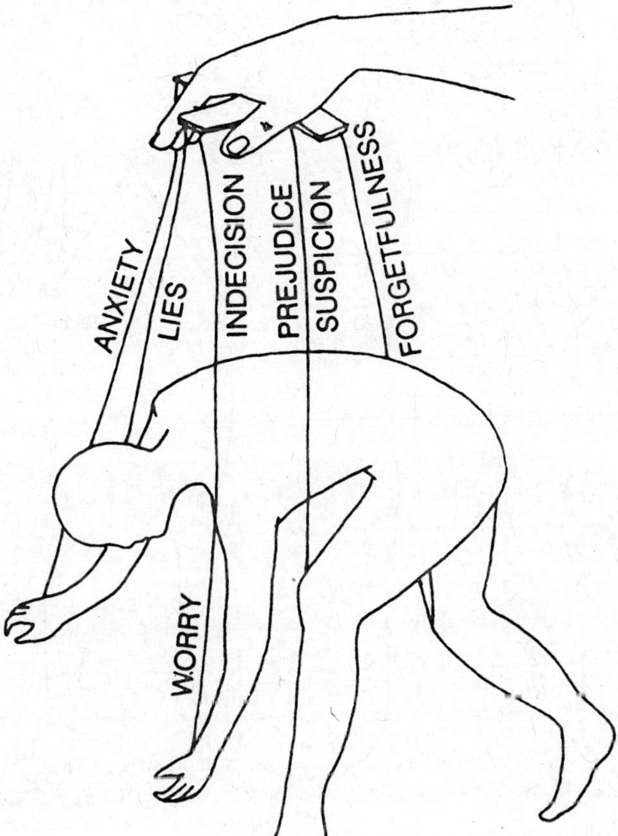

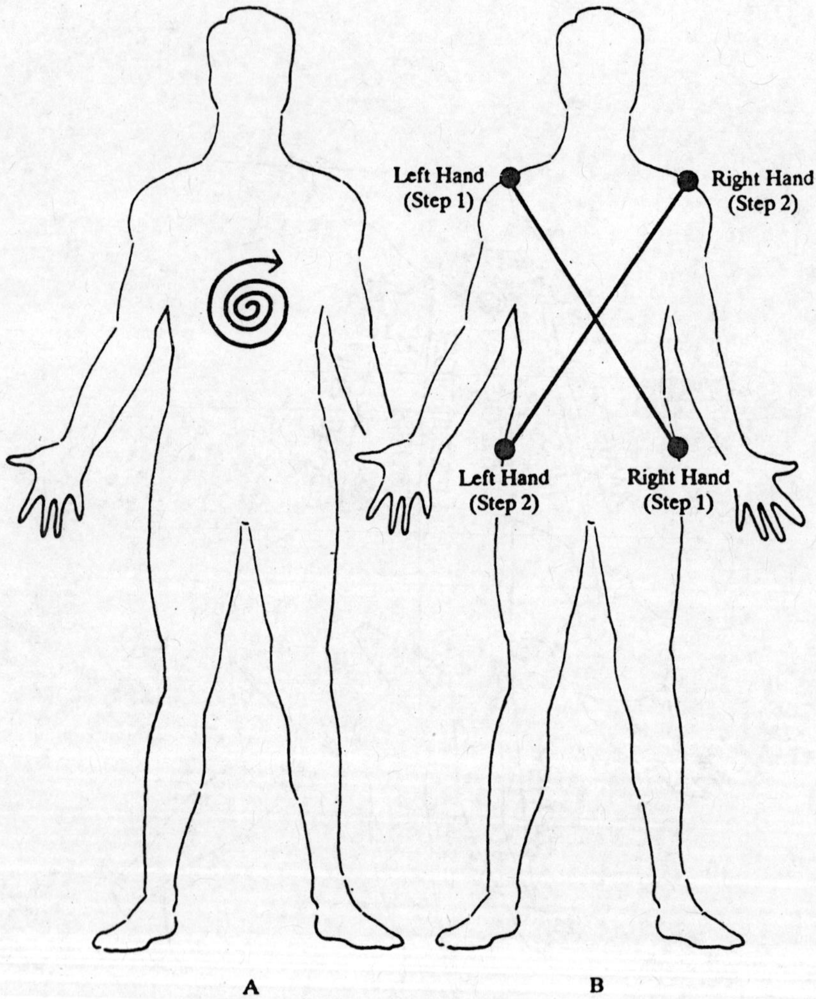

Figure 10. The solar plexus chakra. (A) shows the chakra location and (B) shows the balancing points.

Location

The solar plexus center is located in the chest area. To assess solar plexus energies, suspend the pendulum directly over the diaphragm muscle, at the V-shaped area between the ribs (see figure 10A, front view). Balance treatment points are also located on the front of the body. To realign solar plexus energies, use the pulse points described under "Polarity Therapy Treatment Points" and see figure 10B.

Developmental Challenge: The Will to Know

The solar plexus chakra is the organic and esoteric center corresponding with the pancreas and spleen. It is the psychological center for the evolution of personal mind, the will to know and learn, and the need to communicate. The solar plexus chakra is the electrochemical accumulator for impressions, memories, conflicts, attitudes and beliefs engendered by our efforts to develop intelligence, and to learn and express ideas, thoughts and dreams. Early negative patterning concerning

- the learning or educational process/environment;
- the status, value, or worth or our intelligence, ideas, thoughts or dreams;
- our right to think for ourselves;
- our manner of speech or communication

will chronically imprint the solar plexus center and create a negative psychophysical feedback loop. The solar plexus center can become temporarily (acutely) disturbed by verbal argument, personal agonizing over decisions, mental strain or overwork (excessive reading, memorization, "cramming" for tests), informational overload, exposure to propagandizing, or mental/ verbal coercion.

Psychological States

Psychological states associated with solar plexus disturbance are paranoia, apprehension, worry, mental anxiety or agitation, obsessive or intrusive thoughts, absent-mindedness, forgetfulness, poor concentration, memory lapse, inattention, self-doubt, uncertainty, prejudice, bias, mental rigidity, lying.

Physical States

Those associated with solar plexus imbalances include digestive and urinary tract disorders, sinus and allergy-like sensitivities, skin disorders, blood sugar imbalance, and pancreatic disorders.

Polarity Therapy Treatment Points

To balance, position the recipient supine (lying on the back). Healer is positioned on the right side of the body and places his or her left hand on the right shoulder and reaches across the body, placing the right hand on the recipient's left hip (see figure 10B). The shoulder point is held steady while a gentle rocking motion is started at the left hip. The body may resist rocking at first, but the hip-rocking motion should be maintained until some freedom of movement is established in the hip/pelvis area. Then, both hands are held steadily and quietly until an even temperature and synchronized pulse is sensed in both locations. Healer then moves to the left side of the body and repeats the procedure on the other side, placing his or her right hand on the left shoulder and stretching across the body, placing the left hand on the right hip, rocking and then balancing.

Meridians

Kidney (page 103), spleen (page 105), urinary bladder (page 107), stomach (page 109).

Aromatherapy

Lavender oil (*Lavandula officinalis*), Peppermint oil (*Mentha piperita*). The anointing point is the base of the brain, just above the hairline.

Homeopathic Remedies

Rosemary, Vervain, Windflower, Scullcap, Walnut, Pine, Mullein, Thornapple, Club Moss, Nightshade.

Correspondences

Color: yellow, *Planet*: Mercury, *Vitamin/mineral*: A, sodium & silicon, *Gland*: spleen and pancreas, *Gemstone*: Jadc, *Musical tone*: E.

HEART CHAKRA CENTER

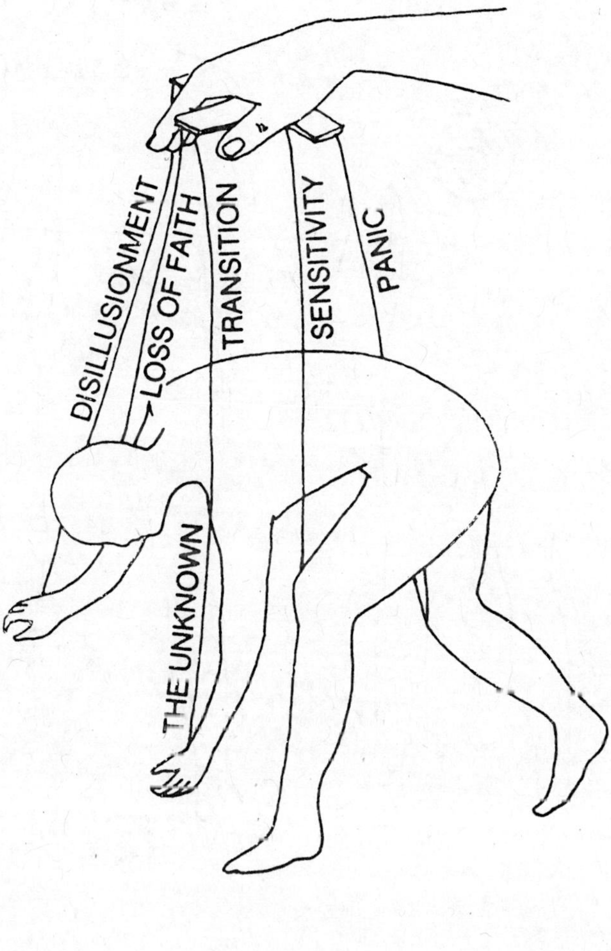

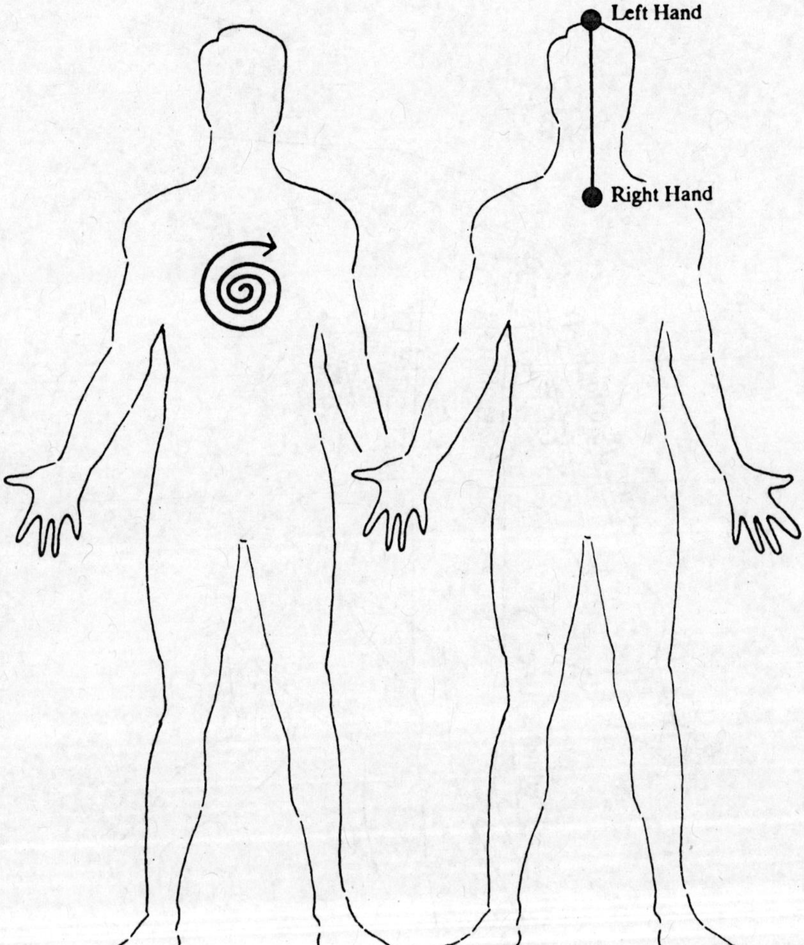

Figure 11. The heart chakra. (A) shows the chakra location; (B) shows the balancing points.

Location

The heart center is located in the upper chest region. To assess heart center energies, position the person supine (on the back) and suspend the pendulum directly over the sternum or breastbone (see figure 11). Balance treatment points are shown in figure 11B and are also located on the front of the body. To realign heart chakra energies, use the pulse points described under "Polarity Therapy Treatment Points."

Development Challenge: The Will to Idealism and Change

The heart chakra is the organic and esoteric center corresponding with the thymus gland. It is the psychological center for the evolution of idealism, the urge for expansion of self-concept and world-view. Included in this developmental area is the need to develop the capacity to love on the transpersonal or universal level. The heart center marks a transition point, the transference point for converting energies from the lower centers to the higher ones. The heart center is almost never found imbalanced unless the individual is undergoing a major transition in the life. If some of the negative attachments to the lower centers have been recycled and released, the lower centers begin to revolve centrifugally and more consistently. The increase in steady, rhythmic energy below the heart center begins to vibrate the heart chakra. A major transition/initiation is usually the result of the shift of energies from the personal to the transpersonal level. As Ram Dass says, "When you hear the sound coming, you have no choice. It slams through your chest and heart. A raw energy surge. The heart is the last overload protection and when it blows, you are free to accept the output of the universe, the radio station that's never off the air."[14] The heart center awakening often places people in the "pilgrim" category, wandering, cut off or removed from all they knew and loved, all that was familiar and comfortable.

Psychological States

Those associated with heart center disturbance are transition disorientation, crisis, euphoria, "trippiness," extreme swings between ecstasy and despair, feelings of loss, separation, numbness, extreme emotional sensitivity, panic.

Physical States

The physical states associated with heart chakra imbalance include exhaustion, "speeding," palpitation, tachycardia, cardiac arrhythmia, panic attack, hyperventilation, flushing.

Polarity Therapy Treatment Points

To balance, position recipient supine (lying on back). Healer places left hand on the very top of the head and the right hand directly over the heart, or breastbone, area (see figure 11B). Hands are held steadily and quietly in place, sensing the pulse and temperature in each location. Hands are left in place until the temperature is even in both locations, and until the pulse is synchronized, beating in unison at both locations.

[14]Ram Dass, *The Seed* (Albuquerque, NM: Lama Foundation, 1974) page 138.

Meridians

In heart center imbalance, check *all* meridians.

Aromatherapy

Jasmine oil (*Jasminum officinale*), Juniper oil (*Juniperus communis*), Hyssop oil (*Hyssopus officinale*). The anointing point is the heart area, directly over the breastbone.

Homeopathic Remedies

Hawthorn, Comfrey, Hellebore, Walnut, Hyssop, St. Johnswort, Monkshood, Ignatia, Leopard's-bane.

Correspondences

Color: green, *Planet*: Jupiter, *Vitamin/mineral*: C and potassium, *Gland*: thymus, *Gemstone*: turquoise, *Musical tone*: F.

THROAT CHAKRA CENTER

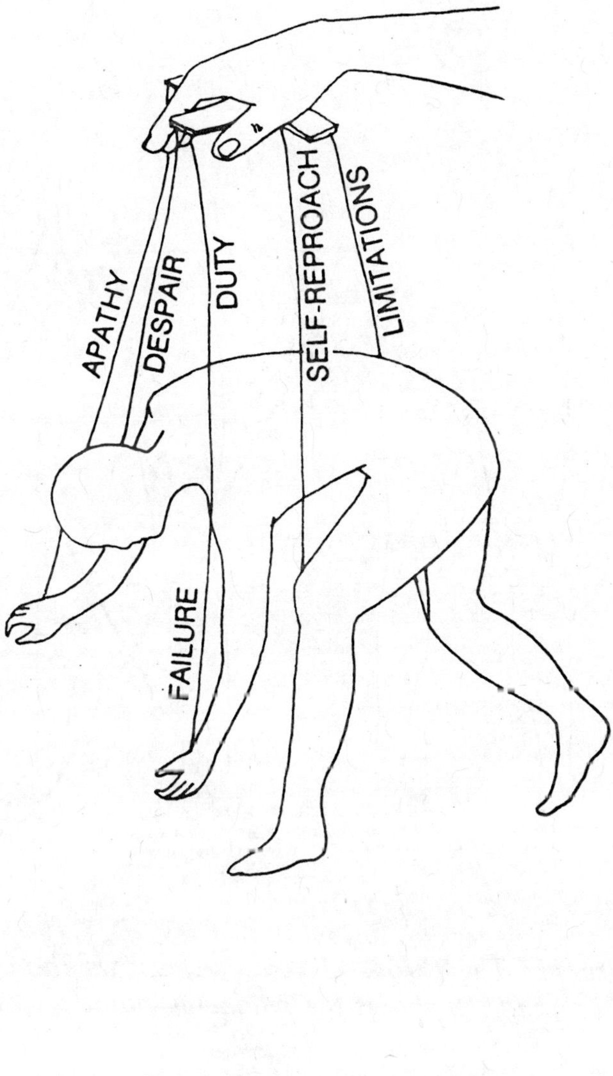

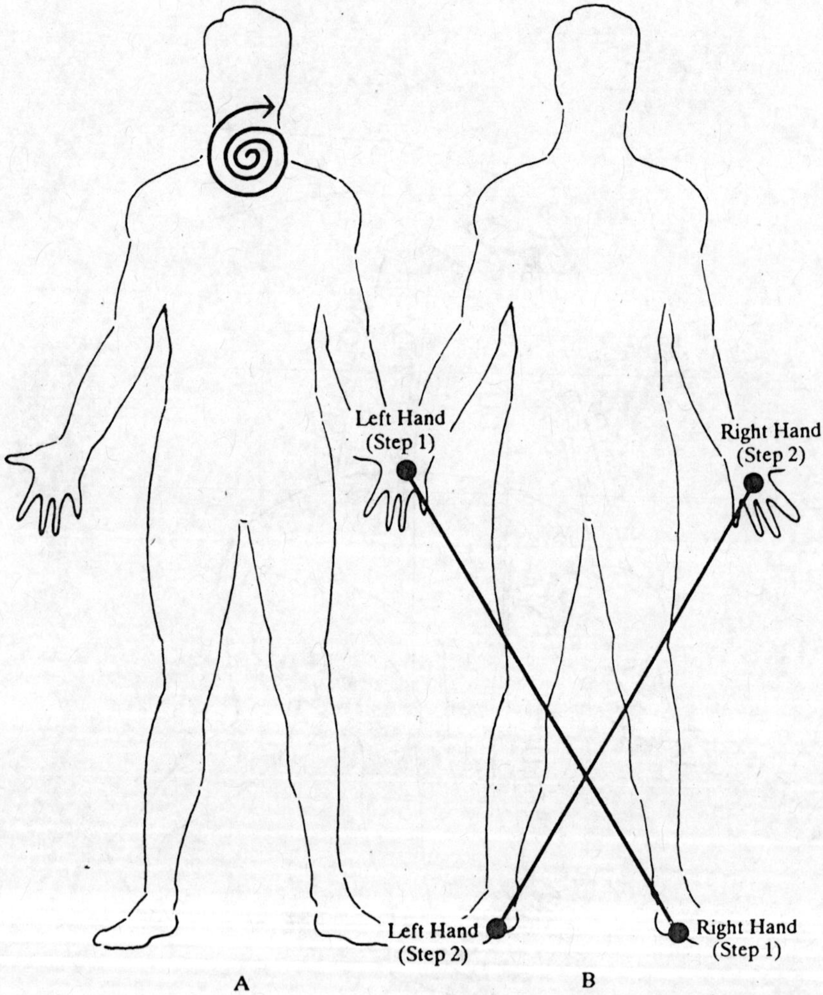

Figure 12. The throat chakra. (A) shows the chakra location and (B) shows the balancing points.

Location

The throat chakra is located in the center of the throat, near the area commonly called the "Adam's apple." To assess throat chakra energies, position the person supine (on the back) and suspend the pendulum directly over the center of the throat (see figure 12A, front view). Balance treatment points are also located on the front of the body. To realign throat center energies, refer to the pulse points described under "Polarity Therapy Treatment Points" and see figure 12B.

Developmental Challenge: The Will to Creatorship and Responsibility

The throat chakra is the organic and esoteric center corresponding with the thyroid gland. It is the psychological center for the evolution of creative focus, self-discipline, initiative and responsibility. Included in this developmental area is the urge to make significant contributions and the need to develop independent and original expressions of value beyond the range of personal recognition and gratification.

The challenge of the throat center is to redirect the energies of the sacral center onto the higher vibratory level, personal work and expression becomes transpersonal building and creatorship. The resonant throat chakra begins to form a resilient bond between the physical vehicle and the Ka body of the conscious mind. The throat center is the chakra of "the word," the vibratory creative force that binds and forms matter. The challenge of the throat center is to master the relationship between thought and form, between mind and matter, and assume responsibility for both content and manifestation of the mind. Trace throat center imbalances and disturbances to the sacral center to discover the source of conflict that is impeding the function and development of the throat chakra.

Psychological States

The throat center disturbances include creative block, "writer's block," fear of success or failure, lack of creative focus or concentration, scattering of creative energy, self reproach, frustration and self-pressuring, fear of creative power or potential, manipulation or misuse of creative will, lack of faith in personal vision, suppressed or hidden grief.

Physical States

Physical states associated with throat center imbalance include lowered immune response, bacterial or viral infection or susceptibility, colds, influenza, herpes, and the like.

Polarity Therapy Treatment Points

To balance, position recipient supine (lying on back). Healer is positioned on the right side of the body. Healer takes the recipient's right hand in his or her left hand; healer's left palm contacts recipient's right palm. Healer reaches across body and grasps the left foot in his or her right hand, sole of foot contacting palm of hand. These pulse points are held quietly and steadily until an even temperature and a balanced, synchronized pulse is sensed in both locations. The healer then moves to the left side of the body and repeats the balancing procedure, taking the recipient's left hand in his or her right hand and stretching across the body to grasp the sole of the right foot in his or her left hand. See figure 12B.

Meridians

Check heart (page 87), circulatory (page 89), triple warmer (page 91), and small intestine (page 93).

Aromatherapy

Eucalyptus oil (*Eucalyptus globulus*), Camphor oil (*Cinnamomum camphora*), Sassafras oil (*Sassafras albidum*). The anointing point is the temples (the sides of the forehead).

Homeopathic Remedies

Wild Oat, Ignatia, Crabapple, Poison Ivy, Windflower, Club Moss.

Correspondences

Color: blue, *Planet*: Saturn, *Vitamin/mineral*: K and iodine, *Gland*: thyroid, *Gemstone*: obsidian, *Musical tone*: G.

BROW CHAKRA CENTER

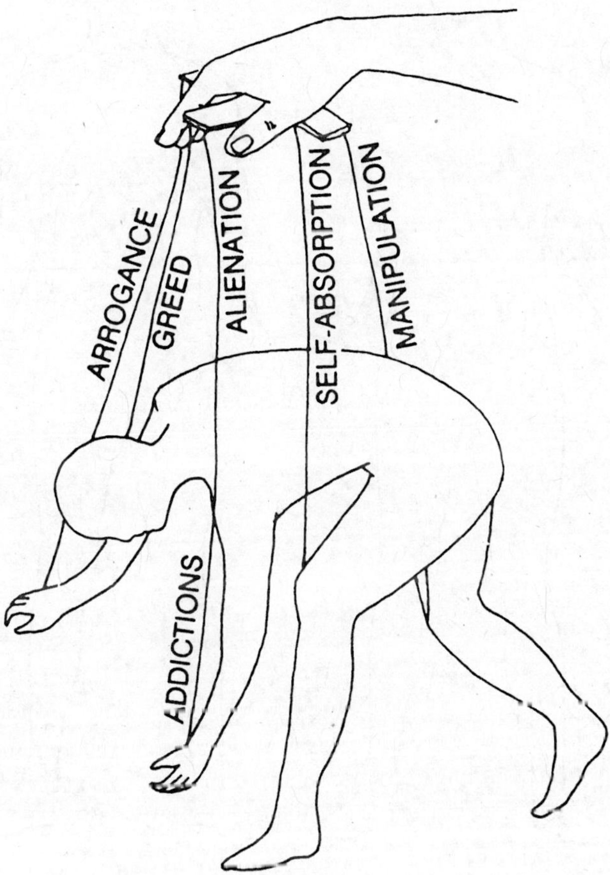

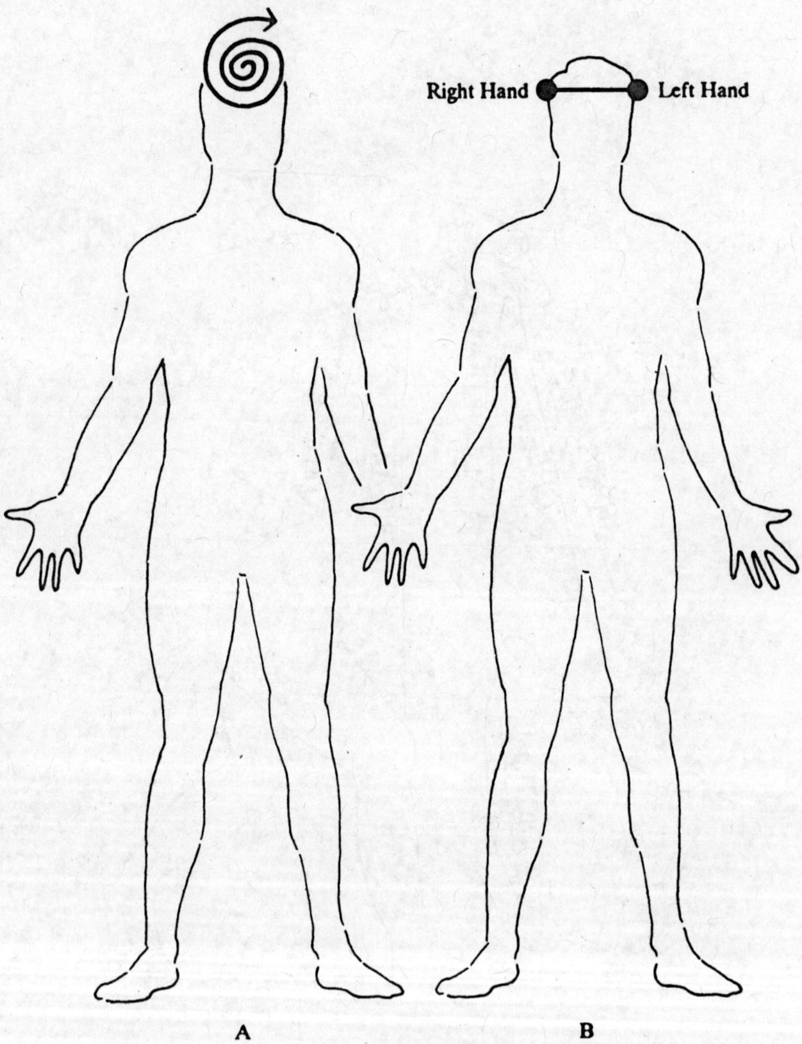

Figure 13. The brow chakra. (A) shows the chakra location and (B) shows the balancing points.

Location

The brow chakra is located in the middle of the forehead. To assess brow chakra energies, position person supine (on back) and suspend the pendulum directly over the forehead (see figure 13A). Balance treatment points are also located on the front of the body. To realign brow center energies, refer to pulse points described under "Polarity Therapy Treatment Points" and shown in figure 13B.

Developmental Challenge: The Will to Leadership and Power

The brow chakra is the organic and esoteric center corresponding with the pituitary gland. It is the psychological center for the evolution of the will to leadership and group integration and the urge for power and control.

The challenge of the brow chakra is to redirect the energies of the personal attraction-desire force (navel center) onto the higher vibrational octave level of charismatic and responsible leadership and stewardship (brow). The resonant brow chakra begins to form a resilient bond between the Haidit body of the unconscious mind and the physical vehicle. Because the brow center opens a channel between the unconscious body and the physical self, a deeper layer of fears, phobias and compulsions must now be confronted and resolved—the fears resident on the unconscious level of being. This is why so many charismatic and emotionally magnetic leaders (recycled and empowered energies of the navel center) become conduits for destruction—

manipulators of power, emotion, money or sex. They use the attracting force of the awakened brow without clearing the debris from the unconscious, resulting in a degrading misuse of the attraction/desire force. Trace brow center imbalances to the lower octave navel center to discover the conflicts that are impeding the function and development of the brow center.

Psychological States

Those associated with the brow center imbalance include superiority, alienation, manipulation, arrogance, aloofness, feelings of power, invincibility, "grandeur," cravings, "binges," substance abuse, addiction, dependencies, self-absorption, greed, persecution, resentment.

Physical States

Those associated with brow center imbalances include substance abuse, dependency, cravings (for food, alcohol, and so on).

Polarity Therapy Treatment Points

To balance, position the recipient either supine or sitting on a chair. Healer stands behind the head and places his or her left hand on the left temple and the right hand on the right temple as shown in figure 13B. Hands are held steadily and quietly in place, sensing pulse and temperature. Hands are kept in place until an even temperature is sensed in both locations, and an even, synchronized pulse is sensed in both locations.

Meridians

Check the lower octave navel meridians: liver (page 97), gall bladder (page 99), lung (page 95), and large intestine (page 101).

Aromatherapy

Sandalwood oil (*Santalum album*) and Cedarwood oil (*Juniperus virginiana*). The anointing point is the temples (sides of forehead).

Homeopathic Remedies

St. Johnswort, Yarrow, Willow, Stavesacre, Holly, Chamomile, Vervain, Mullein, Skullcap, Poison Ivy, Crabapple.

Correspondences

Color: indigo, *Planet*: Uranus, *Vitamin/mineral*: B complex and magnesium, *Gland*: pituitary, *Gemstone*: aquamarine, *Musical tone*: A.

CROWN CHAKRA CENTER

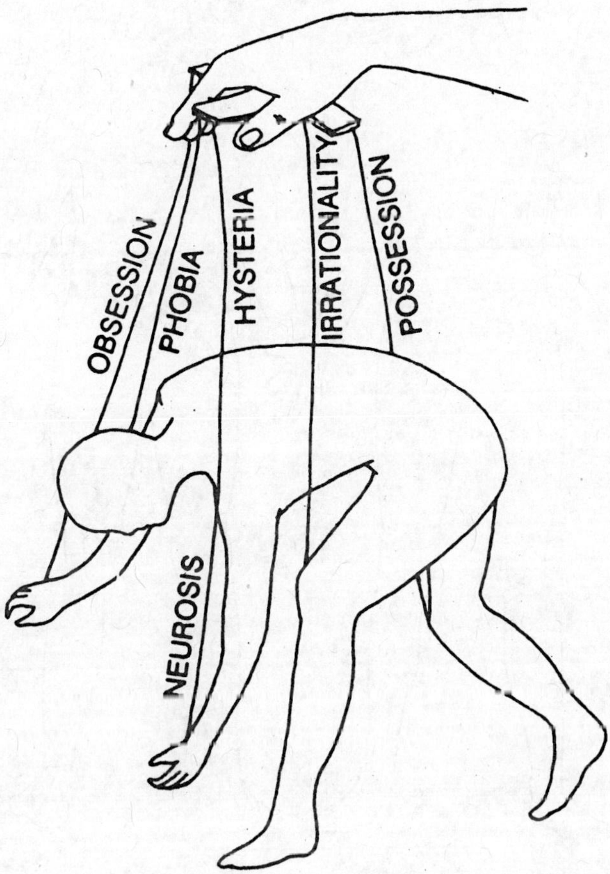

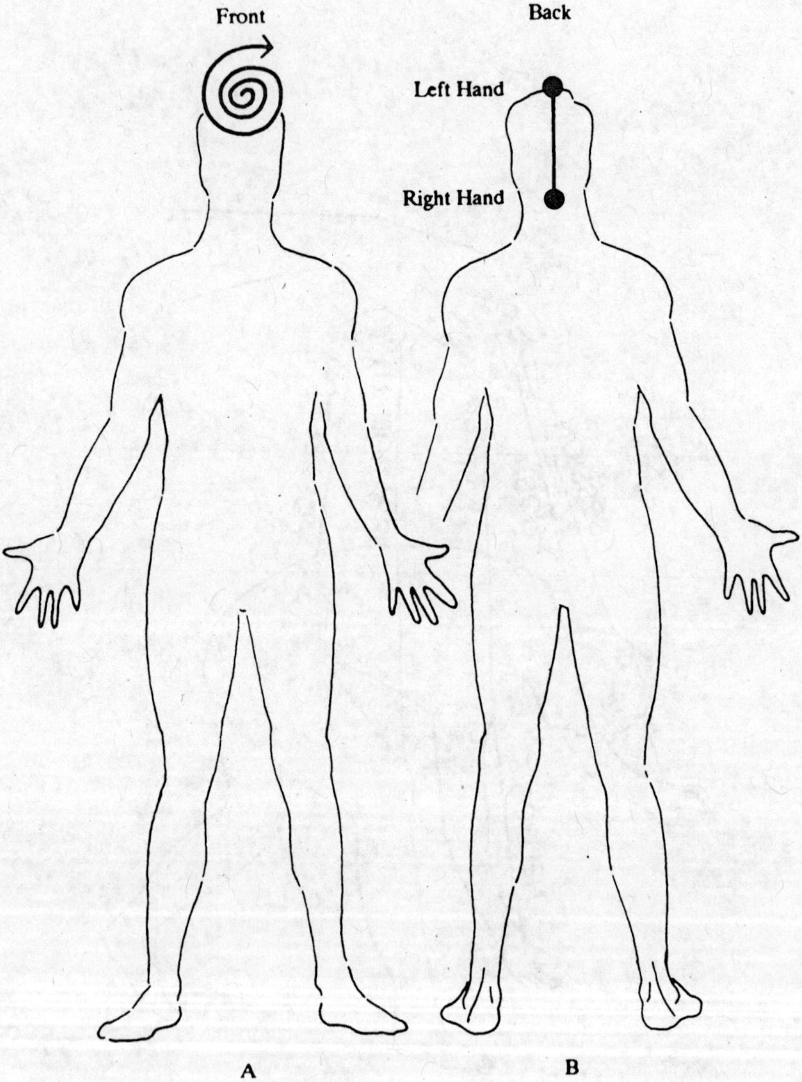

Figure 14. The crown chakra. (A) shows the chakra location; (B) shows the balancing points.

Location

The crown chakra is located on the top of the head, at the fontanelle. To assess crown center energies, position the person supine (on the back) and suspend the pendulum directly adjacent to the top of the head (see figure 14A, front view). Balance treatment points are located on the front and back of the head. To realign crown center energies, refer to the pulse points described in "Polarity Therapy Treatment Points" and see figure 14B, back view.

Developmental Challenge: The Will to Service and Intuition

The crown chakra is the organic and esoteric center corresponding with the pineal gland. It is the psychological center for evolution of the will to intuitive capacity, essence experience and self-actualization, and the need for a sense of transcendent unification or personal experience of the divine.

The challenge of the crown center is to redirect the energy of the solar plexus center—personal mind and communication power—onto the higher vibrational level of the crown center—transpersonal mind (intuition) and channelship. The resonant crown center begins to form a resilient bond between the physical vehicle and the Khu body of the collective consciousness. The Khu body is resident on the archetypal level of school-temple, under the guidance of the master teacher. The challenge of the resonant crown center is responsible channelship and a conscious alignment with the higher self. By means of the awakened crown center, one is "in the world, but not of it," and may function as an avenue for grace, healing, and spiritual power into the physical plane. Trace crown center imbalances to the lower octave solar plexus level to discover the conflicts that are disturbing or impeding the function and development of the crown center.

Psychological States

Psychological states associated with the crown center imbalance include susceptibility to psychic-mental aberrations, feelings of "possession" or "psychic attack," disorientation, extreme sensitivity, vulnerability to negative thought forms, phobias, paranoia, hysteria, obsessions, morbid depression, fear of insanity, and irrationality.

Physical States

Physical states associated with crown center imbalance include nervous system disorders, insomnia, neuritis, headaches, hysteria, restlessness, sensory dysfunctions such as hearing loss, cataract, stuttering, and eyesight impairments.

Polarity Therapy Treatment Points

To balance, position recipient either lying prone (on the stomach) or seated in a chair. Healer places his or her left hand directly on the top of the head and the right hand on the base of the skull, at the hairline (shown in figure 14B). Both hands are held quietly and steadily in place, sensing temperature and pulse at each location. When temperature is the same at both locations and the pulses are beating in unison, the hands are removed.

Meridians

Check the lower octave solar plexus meridians: kidney (page 103), bladder (page 107), spleen (page 105), stomach (page 109).

Aromatherapy

Rose oil (*Rosa centifolia*) and Geranium oil (*Pelargonium odorantiss*). Anointing point is the fontanelle, the very top of the head.

Homeopathic Remedies

Yarrow, Marking Nut, St. Johnswort, Tree of Life, Windflower, Club Moss.

Correspondences

Color: violet, *Planet*: Neptune, *Vitamin/mineral*: D and lithium, *Gemstone*: amethyst, *Musical tone*: B.

CHAPTER THREE

Working with the Meridians

The primary function of meridian therapy is to directly affect the energy levels along a meridian circuit and in so doing, to affect the muscles and tissues supplied by the meridian. Meridian therapy consists of either sedating/decreasing meridian energy or toning/increasing it, and there are several techniques for producing these effects. Although meridian therapy is usually considered to be an Oriental form of treatment, nearly 75 percent of the world's population now uses these energy circuits or centers in one form of treatment or another.

Before we make adjustments to the meridian energies, we need to learn how to assess the energy level along any given circuit. How does one determine whether there is too much or too little energy moving along a particular circuit? One method of meridian assessment considers the tone and endurance level of the muscles in the body. Since each meridian reflexes and supplies at least one body muscle, the condition of the associated muscle will indicate the state of the meridian itself. Muscular pain, tension, and contraction that is not directly related to injury or trauma indicates that the associated meridian is overloaded and congested. The associated meridian is "backed up," so to speak, with electromagnetic energy.

Muscular weakness and fatigue, on the other hand, indicates depleted or insufficient polarity force along the related meridian circuit. The associated meridian is drained and does not have access to sufficient electromagnetic energy. There are several ways in which we may identify muscular irregularities. Muscular pain and tension does not usually require any special detective work to locate. We are all aware of where it hurts, where it is sore, achey and stiff. Muscular weaknesses are a little more subtle. Activity can indicate weaknesses and call them to our attention. Perhaps while putting away the groceries you notice that by the time you have emptied the third sack, your arms are tired and shaky from repeated lifting and reaching into the cupboard. The trouble with activity as an indicator of muscular weakness is that when the action is over, you tend to forget about it until the next occasion recalls the feeling of weakness and fatigue. Careful assessment of postural alignment is a better and surer method of identifying muscular weaknesses.

A body in balance is one that is in good alignment, holding no unnatural stresses or tensions. The shoulders are level, the head is balanced, weight held over the central axis of the pelvis and evenly distributed on both feet. Observing the body and its habitual way of being can yield important clues to structural tensions and weaknesses. Good postural assessment (and the resulting effective treatment) is not a matter of luck or "happening to notice." It is a matter of careful attention and awareness. Learn to look and observe carefully and thoughtfully. Note the tilt of the head, the level of the shoulders and manner of the gait. Do the hands, feet and legs turn out at the same angle from the body midline? Notice the curvature of the spine, and so on. Each weakened meridian is accompanied by a muscular-postural "pictures." Postural imbalances are described with each meridian figure and in Table 2 on page 74. Postural pictures identify weakened meridians and muscles and the associated chakra center disturbance. But first you must learn to observe carefully before you can make effective use of this information.

Identifying predominant emotional patterns also helps to isolate meridian imbalances. Emotion affects the body's polarity by indirectly altering the ionic environment of the cells and tissues. The yang emotions, represented by states of agitation and overinvolvement, overload the body tissues with positive (yang) polarity energy, overstimulating the positive polarity circuits and draining or depleting the negative ones. Yin emotions, represented by states of withdrawal and fear, overload the negative polarity circuits and deplete the positive polarity channels. Identifying predominant emotional patterns tells us which polarity value is overemphasized and which meridian circuits will be overstimulated or depleted as a result. After twelve years of careful observation, research, and recording in counseling and bodywork practice, I have defined more specifically how emotion and conflict impact particular meridians and muscles. I have found that meridian disturbances are often accompanied by emotional pictures or profiles as well as postural ones. The emotional profile describes the type of conflict which upsets body polarity and reinforces or reinstates disturbances along a particular

Table 2. Postural Pictures and Imbalances.

Postural Pictures	Imbalances	
	Meridian	Chakra
Head twisted, not level	Stomach	Solar Plexus
Head craned forward	Kidney	Solar Plexus
S-curved neck	Stomach	Solar Plexus
High shoulder	Spleen	Solar Plexus
Winged out shoulderblade	Lung	Navel
Arms/shoulders turn out differently	Liver	Navel
Hands turn differently	Triple Warmer	Sacral
Rounded/sunken chest	Liver	Navel
Abdominal protrusion	Small Intestine	Sacral
Exaggerated lumbar curve	Small Intestine	Sacral
Flattened lumbar curve	Kidney	Solar Plexus
Lateral spinal curvature	Large Intestine	Navel
Rounded spine	Bladder	Solar Plexus
High hip	Circulation	Sacral
Pelvis twisted, tilted	Circulation	Sacral
Buttock fold askew	Circulation	Sacral
Thigh turned out	Large Intestine	Navel
"Knock" knees	Triple Warmer	Sacral
Ankle turned in	Circulation	Sacral
Pigeon-toed	Bladder	Solar Plexus
Duck feet, turned out	Gall Bladder	Navel
Difficulty climbing	Small Intestine	Sacral
Difficulty getting up from seated position	Small Intestine	Sacral
Can't balance on toes	Triple Warmer	Sacral
Flat feet, fallen arches	Bladder	Solar Plexus
Body tilts forward	Triple Warmer	Sacral

meridian circuit. When muscular-postural assessment locates a disturbed meridian, you should check to see if the conflict associated with the meridian represents an emotional issue underlying or reinstating the polarity imbalance. If this is the case, appropriate counseling, homeopathic remedy selection and vibrational therapy can be used to assist in resolving the emotional pattern and restoring balance.

THE SHENG CYCLE

The body meridians are like a river, flowing one into the other. If part of the river is swollen and congested by a log jam, the water level downstream slows to a trickle. The body meridians function in the same way. The Chinese Creation Cycle, called the Sheng Cycle, illustrates how one meridian flows into another. When we locate a weak muscle (and depleted meridian) or a tense muscle (and overstimulated meridian), we can use the Sheng Cycle to learn which additional circuit will also be affected by the disturbance in the meridian river. If we find a tense, painful muscle, we know that its related meridian is congested, swollen with too much energy. We look "downstream" (clockwise) on the Sheng Cycle to find the meridian which will be feeble and depleted as a result of the energy jam upstream. Conversely, if we locate a weak muscle, we know that its related meridian is depleted; we can look "upstream" (counter-clockwise) on the Sheng Cycle to find the meridian that is overstimulated and blocking energy from reaching the drained circuit.

The Sheng Cycle tells us how and where to balance and readjust the meridian energies when an imbalance

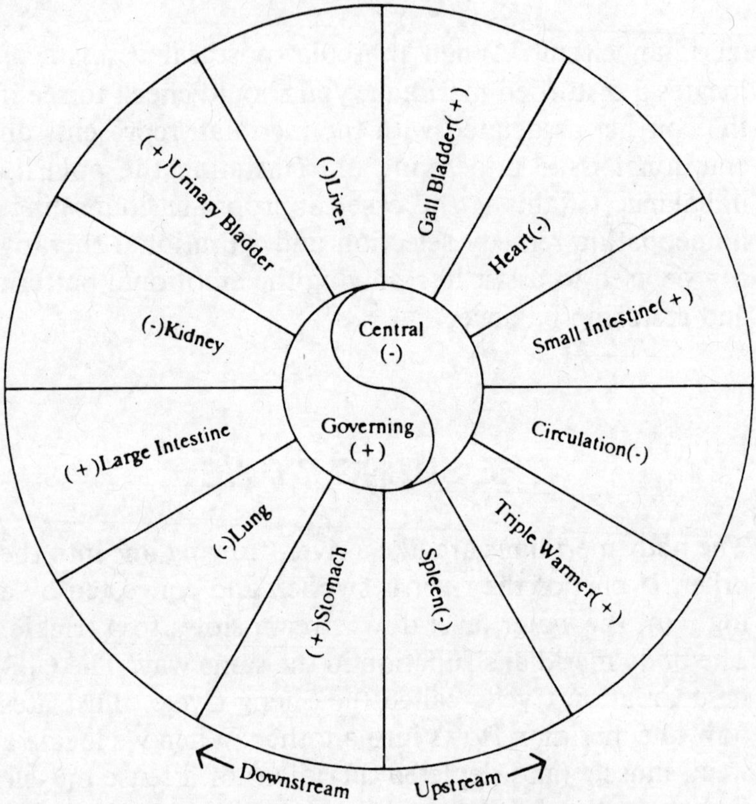

Figure 15. The Sheng Cycle, or Chinese Creation Cycle, illustrates how one organic meridian flows into another in a clockwise direction. The organic circuits also flow from/into the storage circuits, the central and governing meridians, which are shown in the center of the wheel. When a meridian imbalance is located, the Sheng Cycle can be used to learn which additional meridian will also be disturbed. A congested meridian will weaken the adjacent clockwise (downstream) circuit. Or, if a weakened meridian is located, the adjacent counterclockwise (upstream) meridian will be overstimulated. The polarity value of each of the organic circuits is indicated (–) yin-negative and (+) yang-positive.

has been located. For example, if we find the neck muscles to be tense, sore, and stiff, we know that their meridian supplier—the stomach circuit—is congested and overstimulated. We look downstream on the Sheng Cycle to discover which meridian will be drained and depleted as a result. The Sheng Cycle tells us that the lung meridian is being drained and deprived of proper energy flow if the stomach meridian is overstimulated. In balancing, we work with both circuits; sedating the overstimulated stomach meridian and toning the weakened lung circuit and tissues.

There are basically two effects that can be achieved through meridian therapy. Energy along a meridian channel can be sedated/decreased or it can be toned/increased. There are several methods of readjusting the meridian energies

Myotherapy (muscle massage)
Pressure Pointing, and
Meridian Tracing.[15]

When a muscle is sedated and relaxed, electrical energy along its related meridian circuit is decreased. On the other hand, if we tone a muscle and cause it to contract, energy along the muscle's meridian is increased. Changing a muscle state changes the state of its related meridian. Skeletal muscles produce movement by exerting force on tendons, which in turn, pull on bones. Usually the point of attachment of the muscle-tendon to the most stationary bone is called the muscle origin. The attachment of the other end of the muscle-tendon to the moveable bone is called the muscle insertion. The thick

[15]For a complete description of meridian locations and directions, myotherapy and meridian therapy, see John Thie, *Touch for Health* (Marina del Rey, CA: DeVorss, 1979).

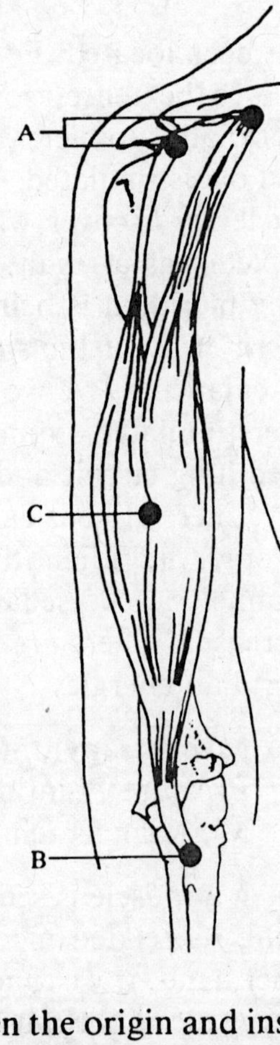

Figure 16. Example of muscle anatomy of upper arm:
(A) points of muscle origin;
(B) points of muscle insertion;
(C) muscle belly or center.

fleshy portion of muscle in between the origin and insertion is called the muscle belly. In producing movements, the bones act as levers and the joints act as fulcrums for the movement of the levers (bones). See figure 16.

Toning a Muscle

To tone a muscle and cause it to contract, place your fingers at the tendon ends of the muscle (points of origin and insertion) where it attaches to the bones. Using medium pressure, juggle or shake the muscle ends back and forth a few times. Next, with firm pressure on the belly or center of the muscle, comb or stretch the muscle out from its center toward its ends. Last, place firm pressure on the origin and insertion points and hold steadily for five to ten seconds. This technique causes a muscle to shorten and contract, and increases electromagnetic energy along the circuit related to the muscle.

Sedating a Muscle

To sedate a muscle and cause it to relax, place your fingers on the tendon ends of the muscle where it attaches to the bones. Juggle or shake the muscle ends back and forth a few times. Next, using steady, firm pressure strokes from both ends of the muscle, push or "bunch" it toward its center (belly) several times. (See figure 17). Finish by placing firm pressure on the muscle ends and holding steadily for five to ten seconds. This technique causes a muscle to relax and lengthen and decreases electromagnetic energy along the meridian circuit related to that muscle. Each of the meridian

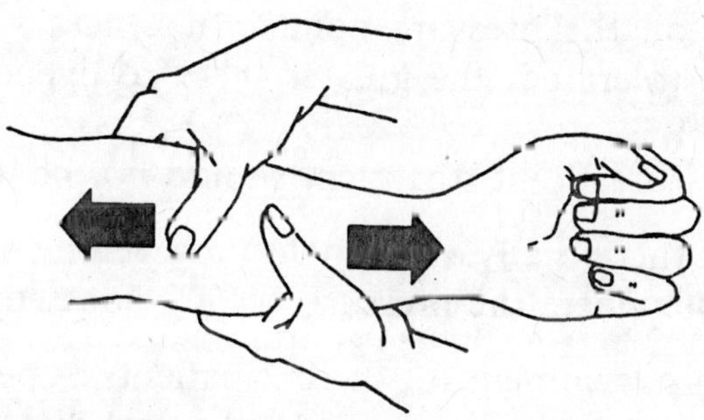

Figure 17. Method of toning a muscle to cause it to contract. The opposite movement sedates a muscle and causes it to relax.

plates illustrates one or more muscles reflexed and supplied by each of the meridians. The action and function of each muscle is also described. For simplicity's sake, each muscle is illustrated only once, on one side of the body. The muscles, however, are bilateral, meaning that they occur on both sides of the body in corresponding anatomical position. When working to tone or sedate meridian muscles, the same techniques should be applied to the muscle on *both* sides of the body, and not just on the muscle illustrated.

ACUPRESSURE THERAPY

Another method used to readjust the meridian energies is called pressure point or acupressure therapy. Use your thumb, or knuckle, to stimulate the pressure points. Small, tunneling movements should be used to work toward a deep, penetrating pressure. Effective treatment consists of 20–30 pounds of pressure held for 1–5 minutes on the pressure points. In general, the more pressure tolerated, the greater the effectiveness of the treatment.

Pressure Point treatment should *not* be used:

- if there is any abnormality or swelling of the skin site where the pressure point is located;
- as a treatment for cardiac patients or people with a history of heart or blood vessel disease;
- during pregnancy or as a treatment for children under the age of seven;

- within one-half hour of a hot bath, heavy meal or strenuous activity.[16]

Each of the meridian figures (pages 87–111) illustrates one or more sets of pressure points which tone and increase the energies of the meridian. These points are used to strengthen weak meridians and their muscles. The pressure points may also be used to sedate the meridian and its muscles. To use the points as sedation points, brush or "flick" your fingers several times over each of the point locations rather than using deep, tunneling pressure. Deep pressure on the tone points energizes and stimulates a meridian and its muscles. Flicking or lightly brushing the tone points sedates and decreases the meridian energy level.

TRACING MERIDIANS

The third method used to readjust meridian energies is called tracing. Tracing a body meridian in its natural direction, from beginning to end, tones the meridian and stimulates/increases electromagnetic energy along the circuit. Tracing a meridian backwards, from end to beginning, sedates the meridian and decreases electromagnetic energy along the meridian circuit. Each meridian is illustrated on pages 87–111. Like the muscles, each organic meridian is illustrated only once, on one side of the body. The meridians, however, are bilateral,

[16]Pedro Chan, *Finger Acupressure* (New York: Random House, 1985) page 14.

occurring on both sides of the body in corresponding anatomical position. When tracing the meridians to tone or sedate a circuit, both the right and left side meridian should be traced.

Identifying emotional patterns and muscular or postural imbalances is the key to locating meridian disturbances. Table 3 on pages 83–84 lists the most common emotional imbalances and the meridian associated with each. Muscular pain, tension, stiffness or contraction is indicative of congestion and overstimulation of the related meridian. Muscular fatigue, weakness and flacidity is indicative of depletion and insufficiency of the related meridian.

If a meridian is depleted, we can *tone* it and increase the meridian circuit energies by:

- tracing the meridian several times in its natural direction;
- placing deep, steady pressure on meridian tone points;
- toning/contracting the meridian muscles;
- sedating the meridian "upstream," or counter-clockwise, on the Sheng Cycle.

If a meridian is overstimulated, we can *sedate* it and decrease the meridian circuit energies by:

- tracing the meridian backwards several times;
- lightly brushing or "flicking" the tone points;
- sedating/relaxing the meridian muscles;
- toning the "downstream," or clockwise, meridian on the Sheng Cycle.

Table 3. Emotional Conflicts & Meridian Disturbance.

	Circulation	Small Intestine	Triple Warmer	Gall Bladder	Liver	Lung	Large Intestine	Spleen	Stomach	Kidney	Bladder	Heart
Anger					●	●						●
Anxiety		●		●					●	●		
Apathy		●	●									
Arrogance								●				●
Bitterness			●		●	●	●					
Competitiveness					●			●				●
Cynicism							●					
Defensiveness					●	●		●				
Depression			●									
Disillusionment			●				●					
Envy					●							
Fear of abandoment				●								
– being alone				●						●		
– commitment										●	●	
– death		●										
– failure	●											
– poverty				●								
– rejection							●					
Grief			●									
Guilt		●										
Hatred					●							
Identity crisis	●											
Impatience								●				●
Intolcrance								●				●
Inferiority	●	●										

Table 3. Continued

	Circulation	Small Intestine	Triple Warmer	Gall Bladder	Liver	Lung	Large Intestine	Spleen	Stomach	Kidney	Bladder	Heart
Indecisiveness									•	•		
Isolation				•			•					
Jealousy					•							
Loneliness				•			•					
Loss of faith			•				•					
Mood swings									•			
Neglect, feelings of						•						
Need for approval										•	•	
Obsessive thoughts									•			
Paranoia		•							•			
Persecution							•					
Possessiveness					•							
Preoccupation										•	•	
Prejudice								•				
Relationship stress					•	•						
Resentment					•	•						
Revenge					•	•						
Selfishness					•							•
Self-pity	•		•			•						
Self-righteousness								•				•
Sexual transition	•											
Shame, regret		•										
Shy, timid	•	•										
Shock, trauma			•									
Victimization	•	•										

If the emotional conflict associated with the meridian disturbance is found to be a part of the pattern of reinstating the polarity imbalance, appropriate counseling, homeopathic treatment and vibrational therapy should be utilized to help resolve the conflict and restore/maintain balance.

Figure 18. Heart: negative-yin polarity circuit.

Location: Begins in the armpit, travels down the inner side of the arm to the end of the little finger.

Toning points: A

Chakra center: Sacral

Muscles: Subscapularis (B) under shoulder blade—turns arm and moves shoulder over ribcage.

Postural imbalance: None known.

Conflict: Self-absorption, self-pressuring, impatience, intolerance, competitiveness, frustration, "do or die" attitude.

HEART MERIDIAN

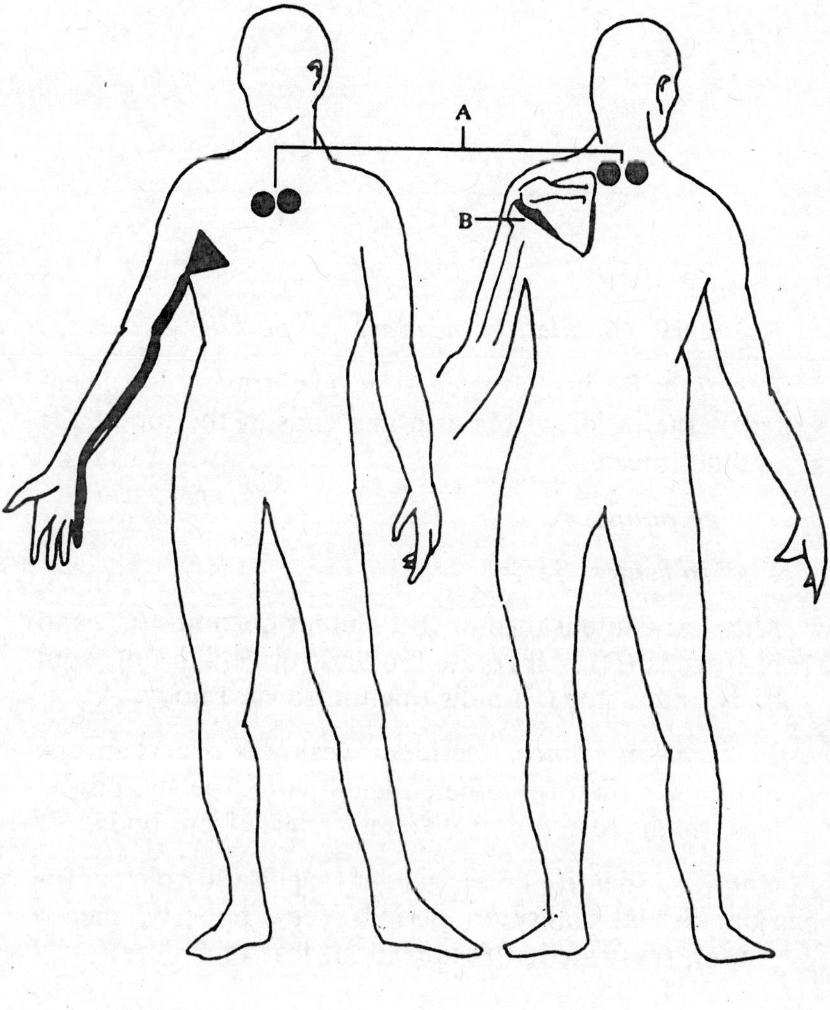

Figure 19. Circulation: negative-yin polarity circuit.

Location: Begins in the chest muscle, travels down center of the inside of the arm and ends at the top of the middle finger.

Toning points: A

Chakra center: Sacral

Muscles: Gluteus medius (B), gluteus maximus (C), and piriformis (D). All rotate hip and turn thigh out from body. Adductor (E) pulls thigh in toward body.

Postural imbalance: Meridian weakness results in one hip higher than the other, tilted/twisted pelvis, bowed legs, thighs turn out at different angles from body.

Conflict: Identity crisis, gender or cultural role confusion, sexual transition periods (*i.e.*, puberty, menopause); frustrated self-expression; fear of failure.

CIRCULATION MERIDIAN

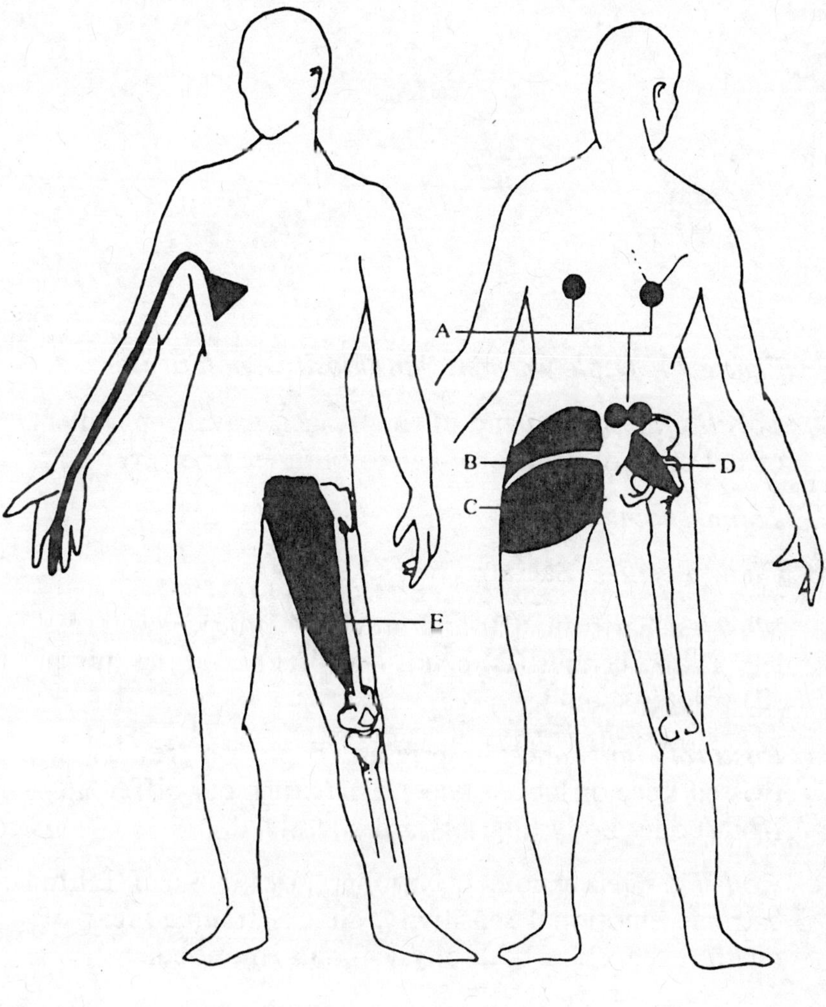

Figure 20. Triple warmer: yang-positive polarity circuit.

Location: Begins at end of ring finger, travels up center of backside of arm, over ear to outer edge of eye.

Toning points: A

Chakra center: Sacral

Muscles: Sartorius (B) and gracilis (C) bend and cross leg; gastrocnemius (D) bends leg, lifts heel; teres minor (E) rotates shoulder.

Postural imbalance: Meridian depletion results in twisted knee or locked knee; hands turn out differently from body; body tilts forward slightly.

Conflict: Depression, mourning, grief, loss of faith; extreme emotional sensitivity, shock, trauma, fear of death; exhaustion both physical and emotional.

TRIPLE WARMER MERIDIAN

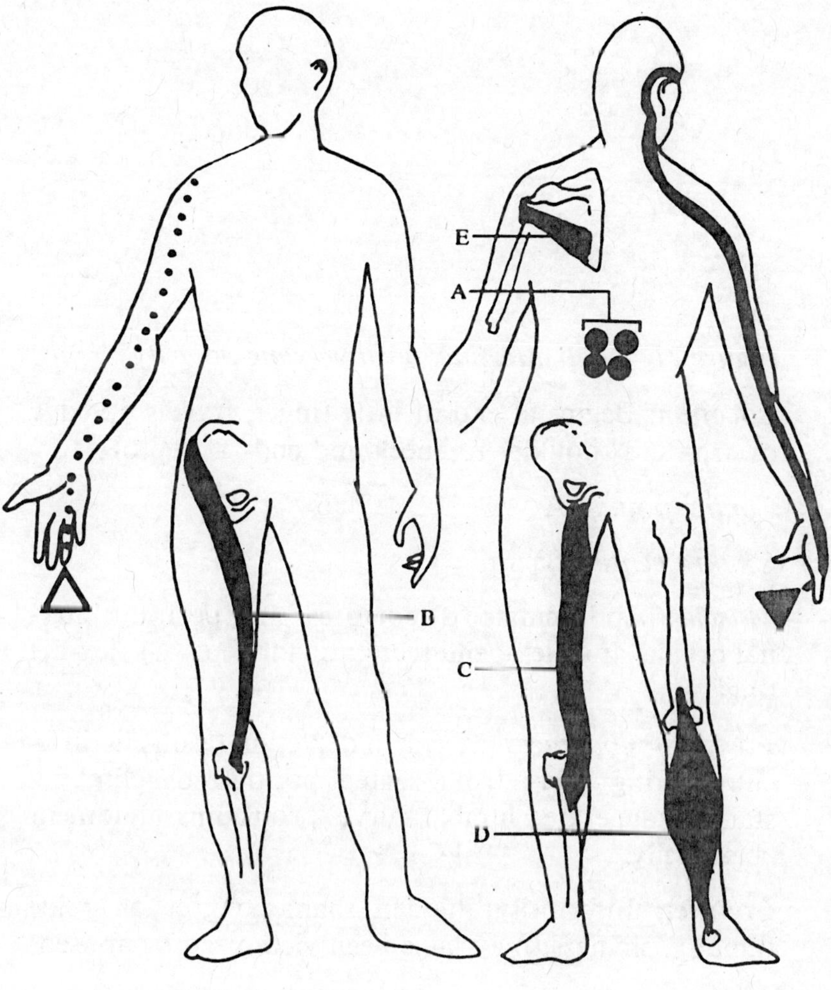

Figure 21. Small intestine: positive-yang polarity circuit.

Location: Begins at end of little finger, travels up edge of arm and shoulder to cheek and ends at top of ear.

Toning points: A

Chakra center: Sacral

Muscles: Abdominals (B) compress and position internal organs and flex-bend trunk; quadriceps (C) flex-lift thigh.

Postural imbalances: Meridian depletion results in difficulty lifting body from seated position or climbing stairs; exaggerated lumbar curve; protruding abdomen, "beer belly."

Conflict: Inferiority; hidden shame, regret or guilt; timidity, shyness; may have been victimized or abused.

SMALL INTESTINE MERIDIAN

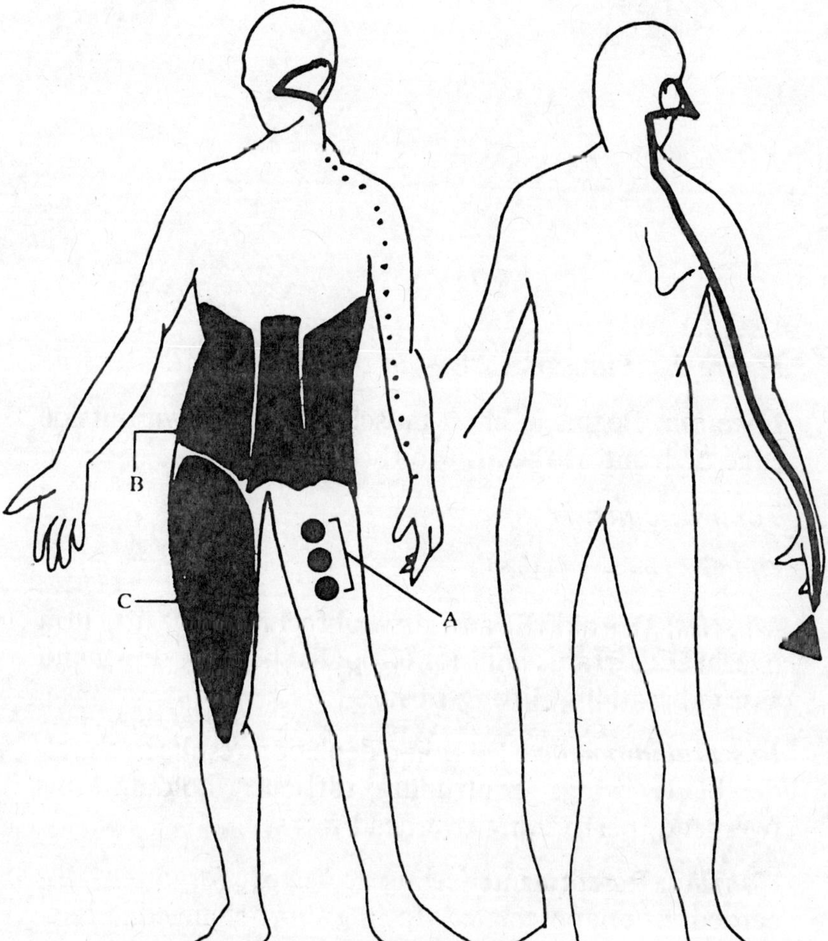

Figure 22. Lung: negative-yin polarity circuit.

Location: Begins in chest muscle, travels down outside edge of front of the arm to the thumb.

Toning points: A

Chakra center: Navel

Muscles: Deltoid (B) and coracobrachialis (D) lifts arm overhead; serratus anterior (C) pulls shoulder down and assists breathing, lifting ribs.

Postural imbalance: Meridian depletion results in shoulder blade "wings" protruding; difficulty holding arms overhead, performing overhead tasks.

Conflict: Resentment; feeling neglected, forgotten, discarded, or unappreciated; feeling short-changed in relationship, giving more than is received or returned.

LUNG MERIDIAN

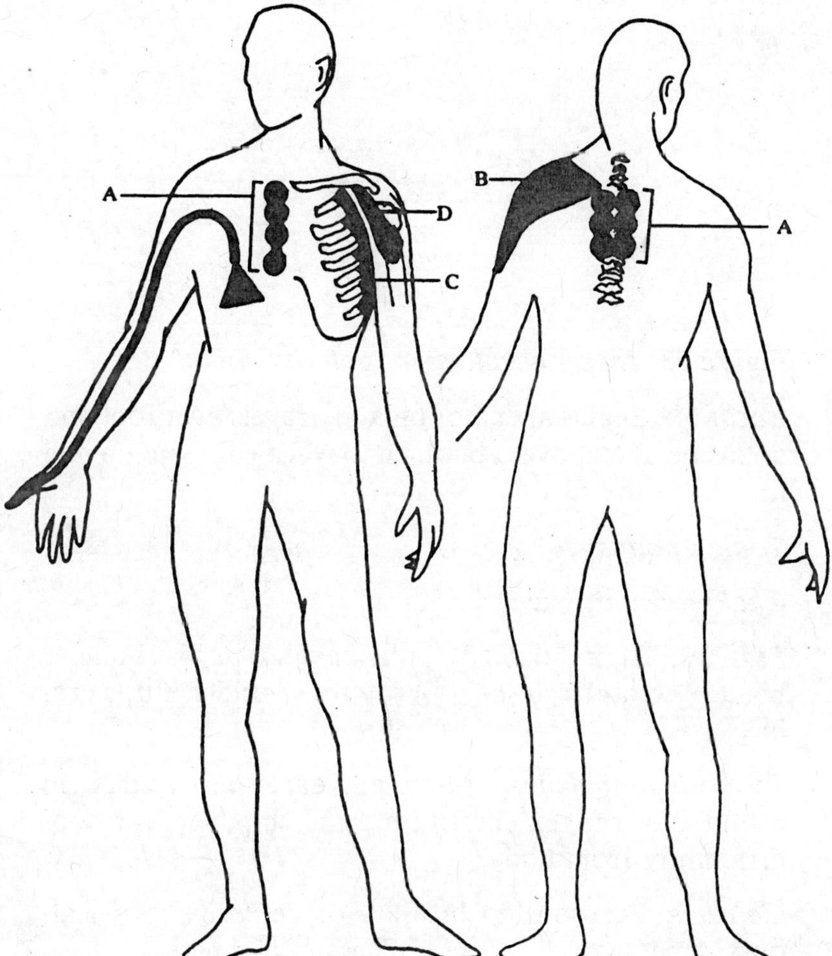

Figure 23. Liver: negative-yin polarity circuit.

Location: Begins at end of big toe, travels over foot and up inside of leg, over abdomen to waist edge and up and in toward the ribs.

Toning points: A

Chakra center: Navel

Muscles: Rhomboid (B) pulls in and turns shoulder blade, pectoralis sternal (C) rotates shoulder, turns arm in.

Postural imbalance: Meridian depletion results in rounded or sunken chest; arms and shoulders turn out differently from body.

Conflict: Relationship hostility or defensiveness; jealousy, envy, hatred, possessiveness, selfishness.

LIVER MERIDIAN

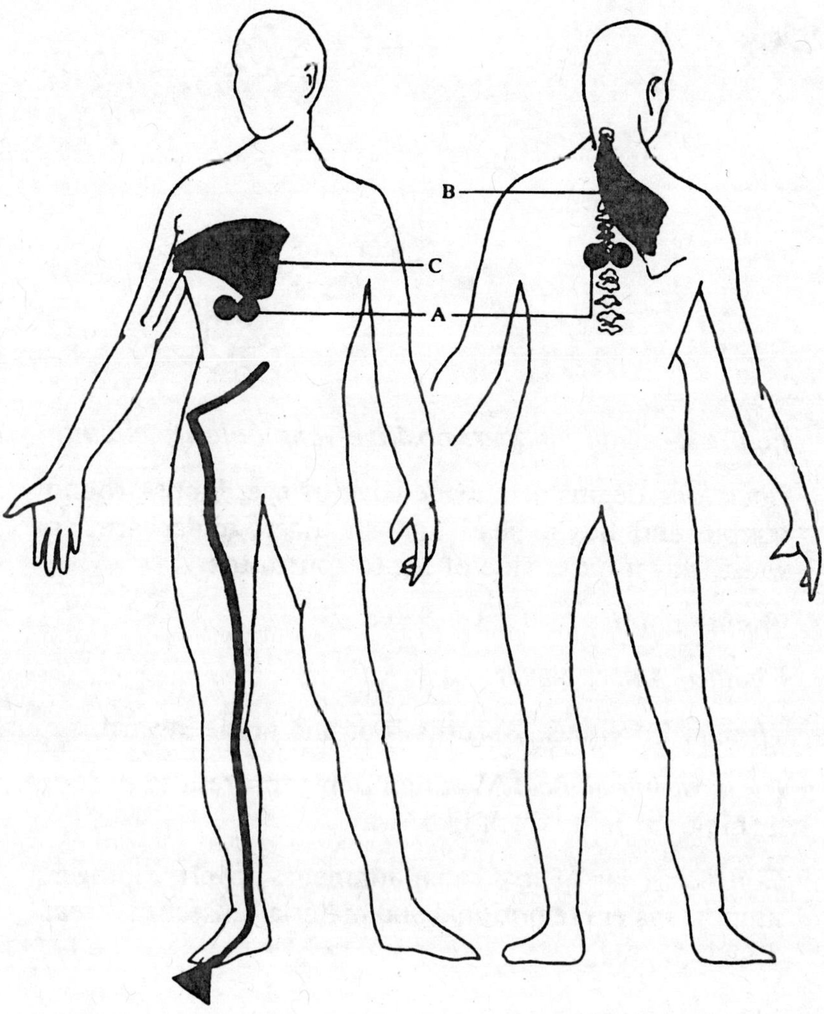

Figure 24. Gall bladder: positive-yang polarity circuit.

Location: Begins at outside edge of eye, loops around temple and down head and shoulder, under arm to waist, down outer side of leg to fourth toe.

Toning points: A

Chakra center: Navel.

Muscle: Popliteus (B) turns foot and ankle inward.

Postural imbalance: Meridian depletion results in foot turning out in a "duck-like" way.

Conflict: Fear of loss, abandonment, poverty, hunger, support system (emotional and material) insecurity, fear of aging.

GALL BLADDER MERIDIAN

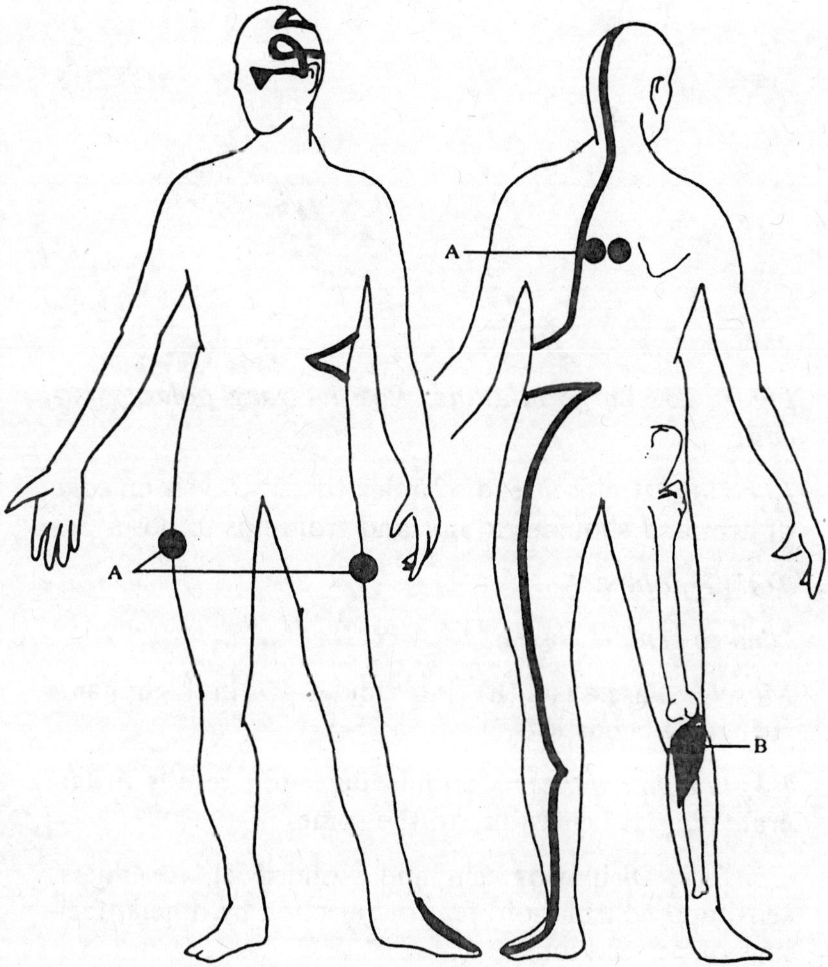

Figure 25. Large intestine. Positive-yang polarity circuit.

Location: Begins at end of index finger, travels up edge of arm and shoulder to lips and from lips to nose.

Toning points: A

Chakra center: Navel.

Muscles: Fascia lata (B) flexes and draws in thigh; hamstring (C) bends leg.

Postural imbalance: Meridian depletion results in lateral, sideways curvature to the spine.

Conflict: Disillusionment and withdrawal, loneliness, self-imposed isolation, fear of rejection by others, feelings of persecution.

LARGE INTESTINE MERIDIAN

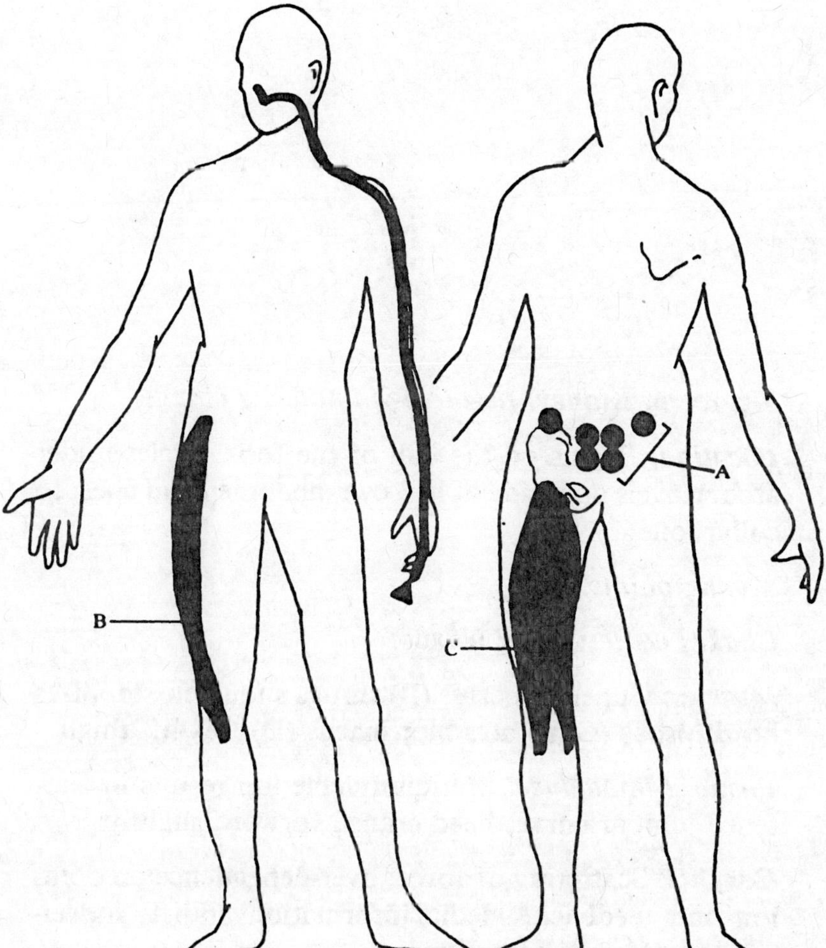

Figure 26. Kidney: negative-yin polarity circuit.

Location: Begins on the ball of the foot, circles under arch, travels up inside of leg, over abdomen and chest to collarbone.

Toning points: A

Chakra center: Solar plexus.

Muscles: Upper trapezius (B) shrugs shoulder, stabilizes head; psoas (C) rotates hip; iliacus (D) flex-lift thigh.

Postural imbalance: Meridian depletion results in flattened lumbar curve; head craned forward slightly.

Conflict: Scattering of force; over-dependence on opinion and feedback; media/information addict; indecisiveness; fear of commitment.

KIDNEY MERIDIAN

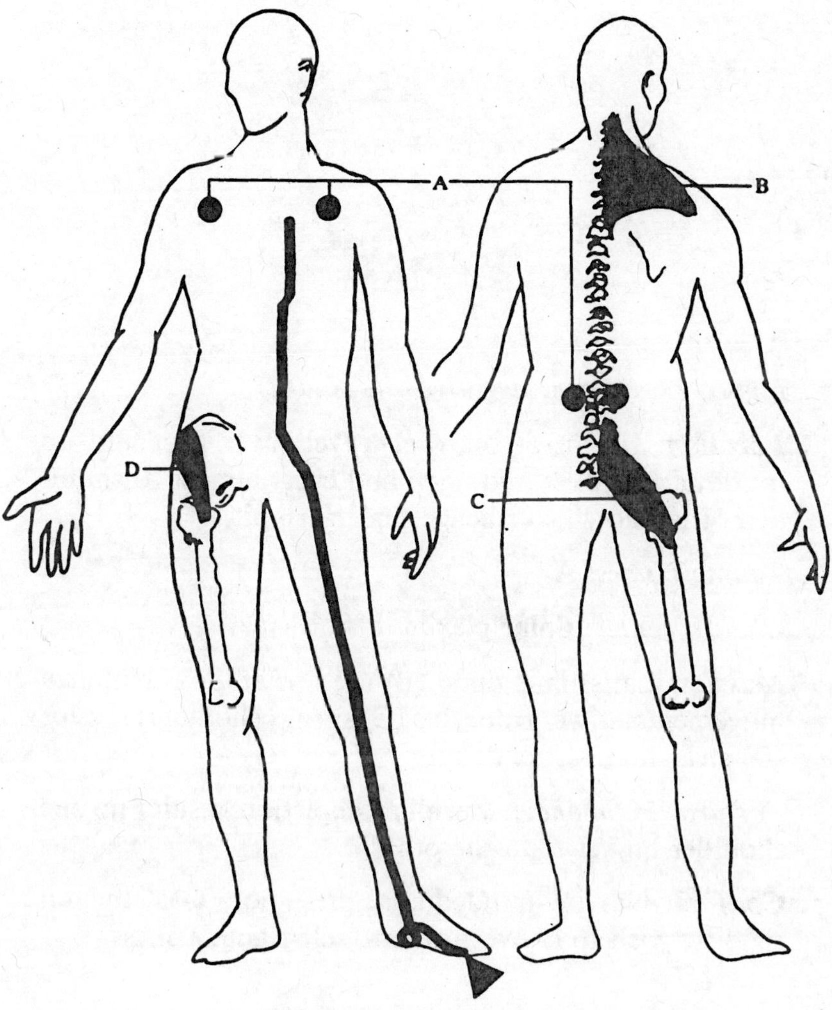

Figure 27. Spleen: negative-yin polarity.

Location: Begins at big toe, travels over foot and up inside of leg, over abdomen and chest almost to shoulders, then down to ribcage under armpit.

Toning points: A

Chakra center: Solar plexus.

Muscles: Latissimus dorsi (B) used in all powerful arm movements; lower trapezius (C) shrugs shoulder; triceps (D) straightens-extends arm.

Postural imbalance: Meridian depletion results in one shoulder higher than the other.

Conflict: Narrow-mindedness, prejudice, bias, mental rigidity, wish to convert others, self-righteousness.

SPLEEN MERIDIAN

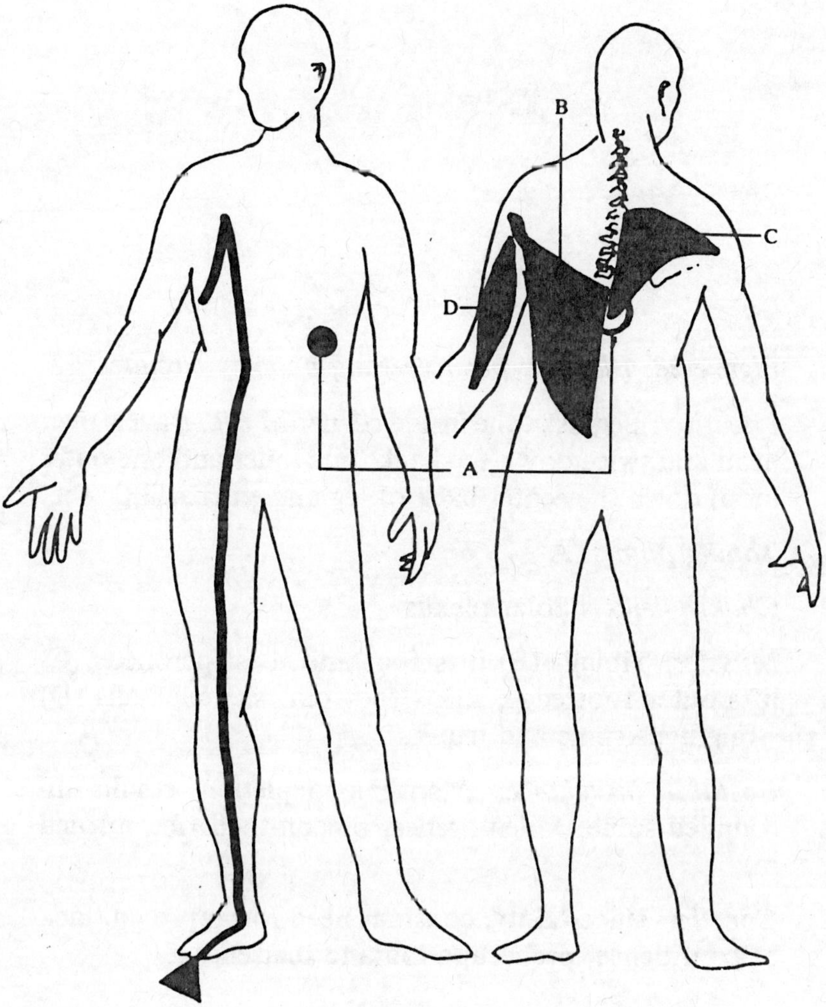

Figure 28. Bladder: positive-yang polarity circuit.

Location: Begins at the inside corner of eye, travels over head and twice down the back (one inner and one outer loop) down the center back of leg and ends at little toe.

Toning points: A

Chakra center: Solar plexus.

Muscles: Tibialis (B) lifts foot and toes; peroneus (C) lifts outer foot edge, turns foot out; sacrospinalis (D) straightens spine and trunk.

Postural imbalance: Meridian depletion results in rounded spine, fallen arches, pigeon-toed (feet turned in).

Conflict: Uncertainty, constant need for approval, lack of confidence, preoccupation and inattention.

URINARY BLADDER MERIDIAN

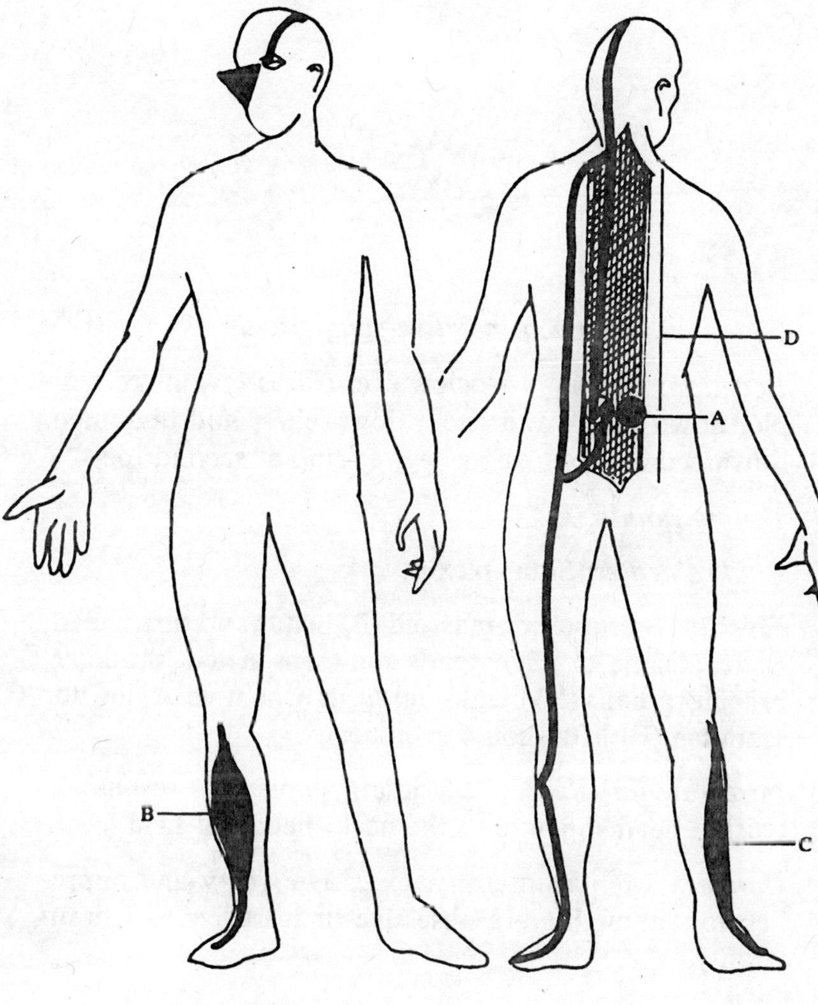

Figure 29. Stomach: positive-yang circuit.

Location: Begins just below eye, traces jawline to temple, down cheek and neck, down chest and abdomen, down center front of the leg, ending at second toe.

Toning points: A

Chakra center: Solar plexus.

Muscles: Sternocleidomastoid (B) bends and turns head; pectoralis major (C) extends and turns arm at shoulder; brachioradialis (D) bends and turns arm at wrist; levator scapulae (E) lifts shoulder blade.

Postural imbalance: Meridian depletion results in twisted head, S-curve to the neck, head not held level.

Conflict: Mental intensity, excessive worry and apprehension, thoughts are obsessive or intrusive and drain vitality.

STOMACH MERIDIAN

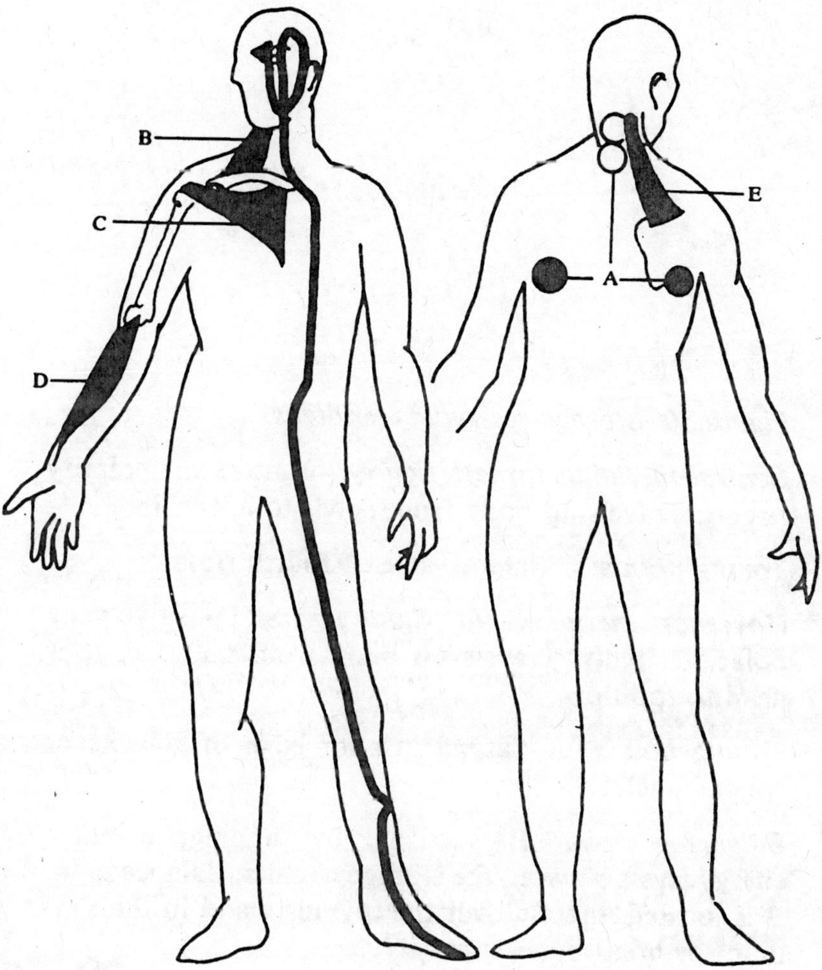

Figure 30. Storage-reservoir meridians.

Central meridian (in left figure): negative-yin polarity circuit. Travels up body from pelvis to lower lip.

Toning points: C (lateral edge of fourth rib).

Governor meridian (in right figure): positive-yang polarity circuit. Travels up body from tailbone, over head to top lip.

Toning points: A (lateral inferior edge of clavicle or collar bone).

Balancing point: B. Activate by tapping; balances energy levels between the storage circuits. Balance point B is located directly over the thymus gland in the sternum, or breastbone, area.

STORAGE-RESERVOIR MERIDIANS

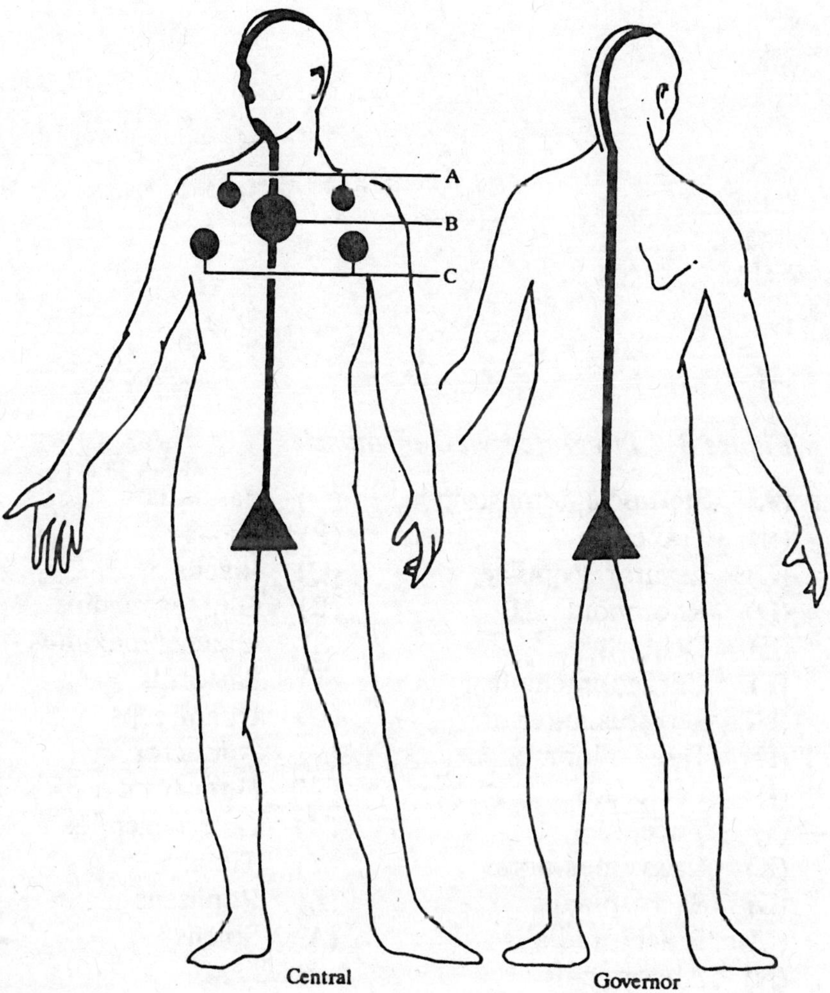

Figure 31. Integrated view of muscles.

(A) Sternocleidomastoid
(B) Trapezius
(C) Levator scapulae
(D) Rhomboid
(E) Deltoid
(F) Coracobrachialis
(G) Serratus anterior
(H) Teres minor
(I) Pectoralis
(J) Triceps
(K) Latissimus dorsi
(L) Sacrospinalis
(M) Brachioradialis
(N) Abdominals
(O) Fascia lata
(P) Psoas
(Q) Iliacus
(R) Gluteus medius
(S) Gluteus maximus
(T) Sartorius
(U) Quadriceps
(V) Adductor
(W) Hamstring
(X) Gastrocnemius
(Y) Tibialis
(Z) Popliteus
(AA) Soleus

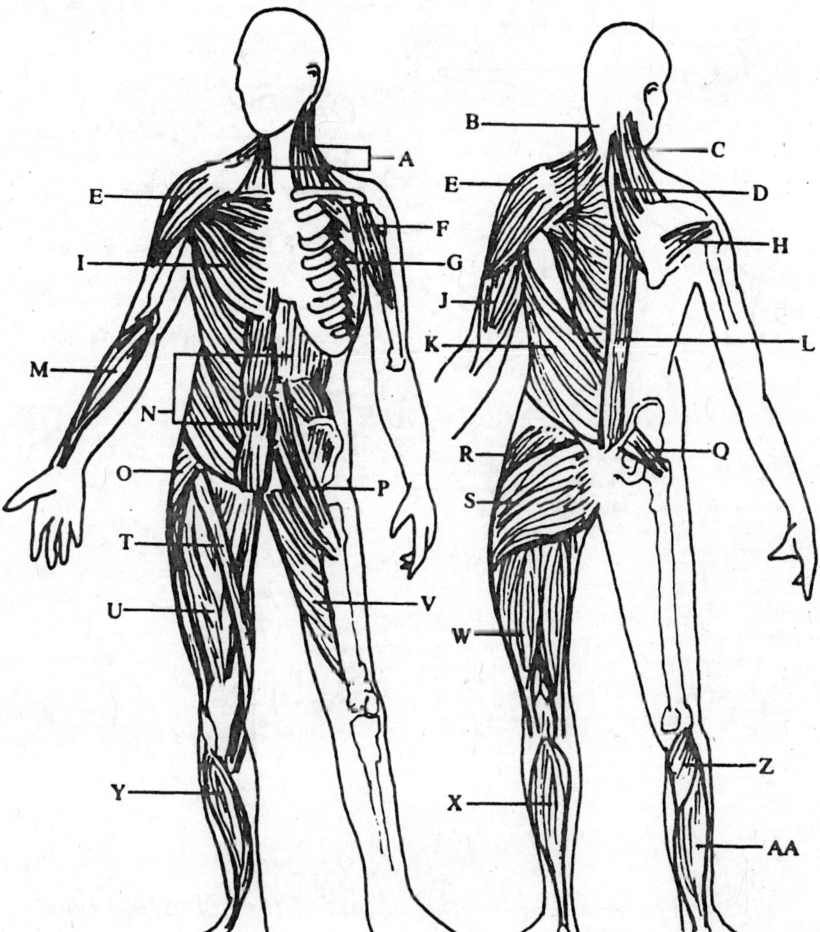
A
B
C
D
E
F
G
H
I
J
K
L
M
N
O
P
Q
R
S
T
U
V
W
X
Y
Z
AA

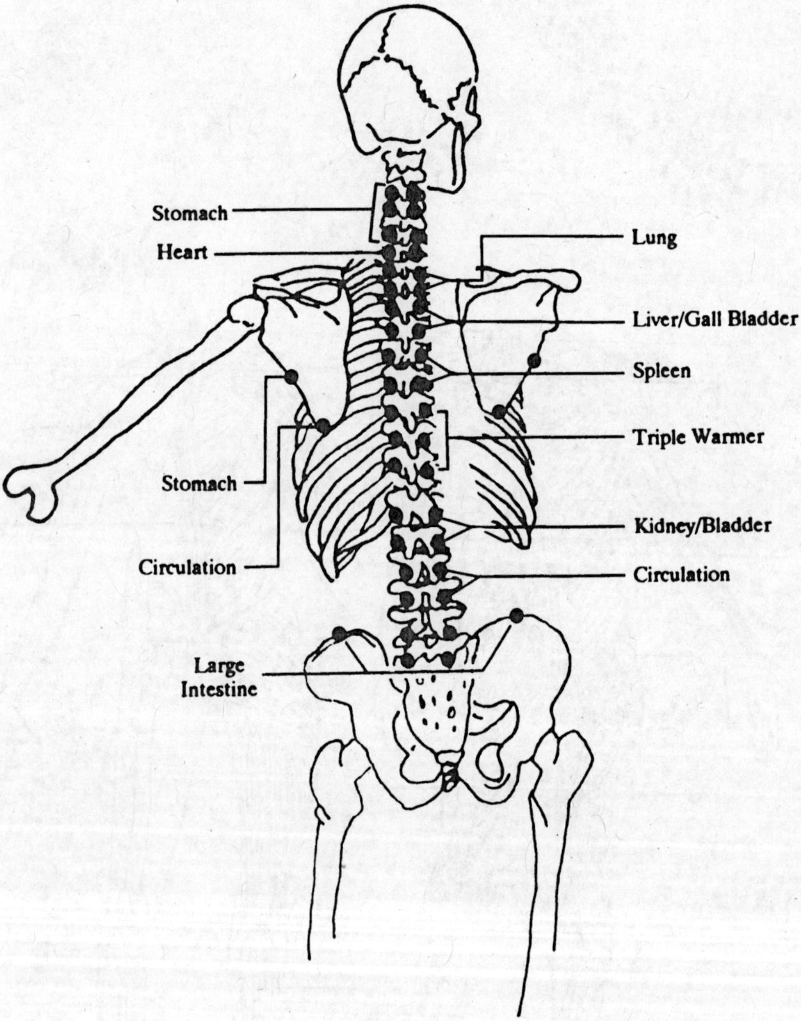

Figure 32. Meridian toning points of the spine and back with reference to bony landmarks.

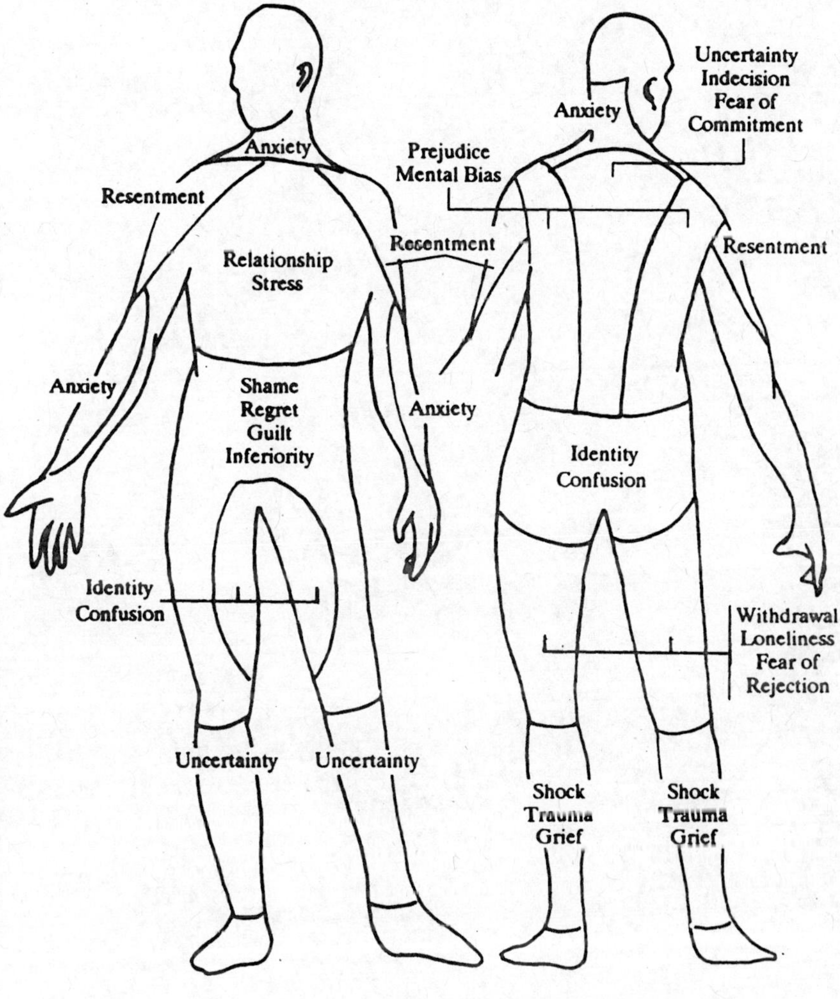

Figure 33. Integrated view of muscular-emotional areas.

CHAPTER FOUR

Vibrational Therapies

The term *vibrational therapy* refers to the therapeutic use of forms or substances that act primarily by altering electromagnetic wave patterns. There is no doubt that our bodies are subtle electromagnetic and chemical realities, governed by polarity law and endocrine microsecretions, as well as the more apparent chemical effects of food, water, movement and so on. It is only in the past few decades that science has developed enough technical sophistication to actually detect hormone and other endocrine secretions in the bloodstream. The field of endocrinology is and will continue to be a major pioneering area for medicine and the other sciences. Advancements in endocrinology have been based primarily on the study of hormone effects, and the formulation and testing of theories about these effects. These two areas—endocrinology and vibrational treatment—are very much interrelated. We are not certain of the mechanics of vibrational therapies, that is, how they achieve the results they do. This understanding is evolving, like endocrinology, from theory and study of the effects of treatment itself.

Some forms of vibrational therapy seem to impact organic electromagnetic wave patterns by directly affecting the body's electrical or ionic environment (polarity and meridian therapy). Other treatments seem to alter wave patterns more indirectly, by means of sound and light frequency (color and gem therapy). Still others may produce effects by impacting the endocrine system itself (aromatherapy) or evoking a complex version of the immune response (homeopathy). We do know that vibrational treatment produces measurable effects, electrically and chemically, which impact both physical and psychological states.

As we begin to learn more in areas of physics and endocrinology, our understanding of the mechanics of vibrational treatment will deepen. In previous chapters we have investigated meridian and polarity therapy, vibrational treatments that directly alter organic electromagnetic wave patterns by changing electrical value and ionic atmosphere. In this chapter, we will explore seemingly more indirect forms of vibrational treatment, including aromatherapy, gem and color therapy and homeopathic remedies.

AROMATHERAPY

The term *aromatherapy* was coined by Gattefosse, a French research chemist of the 1920s; but the therapeutic application of scent predates written history. The word "perfume" is derived from Latin *per* (through) and *fumum* (smoke) and refers to the use of fumigation. "Smoking" is perhaps the earliest recorded form of herbal treatment.[17] Herbal smoking has been employed since ancient times for the treatment of nervous disorders and for the purposes of cleansing and purification.

The sense of smell is unique among human perceptions. Our other senses relay information to neural receptors, which in turn, convey information to the brain. In olfaction (smell), the sensory nerve endings actually protrude through the inner lining of the nose, resulting in direct contact between stimulus and receptor cell. Aromatic stimulation produces an immediate, direct effect on the brain and nervous system.

Odors emit vibrations which can be placed on the electromagnetic scale. Odor perception is a result of both the molecular-chemical structure of the stimulus and of its vibrational rate.

The aromatic quality of a plant is a constituent of its volatile oil, or essence. Essential oils are complex, containing alcohols, esters, aldehydes, ketones and terpenes. A plant's essential oil is unique; it is like it's voice. As Tisserand puts it, "The essential oil is the most ethereal and subtle part of a plant, and its therapeutic action takes place on a higher, more subtle level than that of the whole plant or its extract, having in general a more pronounced effect on the mind and emotions than herbal medicines. The properties of herbs and their essential oils may be much the same, but the therapeutic action is different."[18]

Essential oils are usually extracted by distillation. The amount and quality of the oil yield depends on the plant itself, the climate and soil conditions, and the

---

[17]For in-depth treatment of the history and therapeutic uses of essential oils, see Robert Tisserand, *Aromatherapy* (Rochester, VT: Inner Traditions, 1977), page 17.

[18]Tisserand, *Aromatherapy*, page 10.

time, season, and method of harvest. Heat, light, air and moisture have a damaging effect on essential oils. Oils should be kept in dark-colored, well-stoppered bottles in cool, dry locations to preserve their qualities. Therapeutic use of essential oils should be confined to one oil at a time. Aromatherapy produces both psychological and physiological effects and there are several forms of application used to achieve these effects.

Anointing is the form of application used to stimulate the glandular centers (chakras). Each chakra is associated with one or more oils which resonate sympathetically and electrochemically with the chakra's energy and facilitate the release of congestions and accumulations at the chakra level. In using anointing to stimulate a chakra center, one to two drops of undiluted essential oil is applied to the chakra's reflex anointing point. Anointing may also be used to treat a variety of physical and psychological states, and in such cases one to two drops of the selected oil is applied in undiluted form to the wrists, palms or soles of the feet where it will be readily absorbed by the bloodstream and conveyed to the glands and tissues of the body.

Local Baths (hand or foot baths; also local wet compress applications) are used primarily to treat physical disorders. Add 10–15 drops of the selected essential oil to a small basin of hot water and immerse hands or feet for 15–30 minutes in the solution. Hot water immersion aids in skin penetration and the absorption of the essence's active properties into the bloodstream.

Massage application is also used mainly to treat physical disorders. The therapeutic properties of the plant essence is absorbed through the skin and into the bloodstream, which conveys them to the body's tissues and organs. For massage application, essential oils are diluted in a vegetable oil base. Any good quality oil such as safflower, sunflower, olive, or almond oil may be used. Since oil mixtures can easily become rancid, only the amount to be used should be prepared. To prepare enough massage oil blend for one treatment: pour 1/4 cup (2 oz) vegetable oil into a small bottle. Add 10–12 drops of the selected essential oil and shake well.

In this section I have described seventeen essential oils, the chakra each oil reflexes, the chakra anointing points, and also indications for physical and psychological use.

Basil (*Ocymum basilicum*)

Chakra: sacral
Chakra anointing point: skull base
Psychological indications: depression, melancholy.
Physical indications: paralysis; exhaustion; poor circulation; congestion, colds.

Camphor (*Cinnamomum camphora*)

Chakra: throat
Chakra anointing point: temples
Psychological indications: balances both yin and yang states.
Physical indications: viral and fungal infections: herpes, ringworm, athlete's foot; respiratory disorders, such as cough, bronchitis, emphysema, asthma; pain, neuritis.

Cedarwood (*Juniperus virginiana*)

Chakra: brow
Chakra anointing point: temples.
Psychological indications: fear of loss, aging, self-consciousness concerning image or appearance.
Physical indications: respiratory disorders, such as cough, bronchitis and the like; skin disorders and injuries, such as burns, wounds, rashes, bites, stings.

Chamomile (*Anthemis nobilis*)

Chakra: navel
Chakra anointing point: brow
Psychological indications: irritability, anger, agitation, resentment, relationship stress.
Physical indications: menstrual and reproductive system disorders, painful, difficult menses, menopause; muscle and joint injuries or pain; skin disorders or injuries, such as burns, wounds, rashes.

Clove (*Caryophyllus aromaticus*)

Chakra: sacral
Chakra anointing point: skull base
Psychological indications: apathy, lethargy, timidity.
Physical indications: applied locally for dental pain; digestive disorders such as dyspepsia, flatulence, nausea; poor circulation.

Eucalyptus (*Eucalyptus globulus*)

Chakra: throat
Chakra anointing point: temples.
Psychological indications: shame, guilt, contamination, regret.
Physical indications: bacterial and viral infections; respiratory and throat disorders; colds, flu; wounds and infected skin injuries.

Geranium (*Pelargonium odorantissimum*)

Chakra: crown
Chakra anointing point: fontanelle
Psychological indications: nervous tension, insomnia, negative or obsessive thoughts.
Physical indications: eye and skin wounds, rashes or injuries; neuralgia and pain.

Hyssop (*Hyssopus officinale*)

Chakra: heart
Chakra anointing point: sternum
Psychological indications: hysteria, shock, grief, trauma, mourning, disorientation.
Physical indications: cardiac irregularities, high or low blood pressure; skin wounds or disorders; respiratory problems such as cough, bronchitis, emphysema.

Jasmine (***Jasminum officinale***)

Chakra: heart
Chakra anointing point: sternum
Psychological indications: hypersensitivity, depression.
Physical indications: menstrual and reproductive problems, menstrual pain, hormone imbalance, menopause.

Juniper (***Juniperus communis***)

Chakra: heart
Chakra anointing point: sternum
Psychological indications: fear, trembling, loss of faith or courage.
Physical indications: urinary tract disorders; systemic toxicity, systemic deposits and poisons; gout, arthritis, pH imbalance, tissue acidity; skin wounds and disorders.

Lavender (***Lavandula vera***)

Chakra: solar plexus
Chakra anointing point: skull base
Psychological indications: nervousness, agitation, mental delusion, mental extremes, panic.
Physical indications: skin wounds, injuries or disorders, insect bites; digestive disorders; migraine headaches.

Neroli (*Citris vulgaris*)

Chakra: sacral
Chakra anointing point: skull base
Psychological indications: depression, shock, trauma, accident.
Physical indications: skin rashes, wounds, infection, burns; digestive problems: nausea, dyspepsia.

Peppermint (*Mentha piperita*)

Chakra: solar plexus
Chakra anointing point: skull base.
Psychological indications: confusion, indecision, poor concentration, preoccupation, lack of mental clarity and focus.
Physical indications: neuralgia, neuritis, pain, headache; digestive disorders such as dyspepsia, nausea, motion sickness.

Rose (*Rosa centifolia*)

Chakra: crown
Chakra anointing point: fontanelle
Psychological indications: cravings, appetites, anger, arrogance.
Physical indications: eye and skin wounds, rashes or injury, burns, bruises, bites; reproductive system problems.

Sandalwood (*Santalum albidum*)

Chakra: brow
Chakra anointing point: temples
Psychological indications: nervous tension, apprehension, phobia, compulsion, nightmare.
Physical indications: urinary tract disorders; respiratory disorders such as asthma, bronchitis; liver and gall bladder congestion.

Sassafras (*Sassafras albidum*)

Chakra: throat
Chakra anointing point: temples
Psychological indications: inhibited or blocked self-expression, creative block, scattering of force, lack of priority of creative focus.
Physical indications: respiratory disorders; urinary tract disorders.

Wintergreen (*Gaultheria procumbens*)

Chakra: navel
Chakra anointing point: brow
Psychological indications: emotional and/or relationship insecurity, loneliness, feeling neglected or forgotten.
Physical indications: muscular, joint, and arthritis pain; headaches; cold congestion, sinus.

COLOR AND GEMSTONE THERAPY

We perceive different wavelengths of light as color. Color perception is a manifestation of both light frequency-oscillation and wavelength. Although theories about the therapeutic qualities of color have been scoffed at, few deny the experience of both physical and psychological states associated with color. Color colloquialisms such as "seeing red" and "feeling blue" attest to such associations. Although chromotherapy (color healing) has its roots in the ancient past, it was probably Dr. D. P. Ghadiali's research published in 1933 (*The Spectro Chromemetry Encyclopedia*) that brought color therapy to modern attention. Ghadiali's theory states that colors represent chemical potencies in higher vibrational octaves, and he utilized scientific method to test and explain the therapeutic effects of the spectrum. According to these theories, the therapeutic action of color is an effect of light and vibration. Gemstones, in a way, are a solidified form of colored light, and act as reflectors of specific light wavelengths. As white light enters a gemstone and passes through it, the light is affected by the structural and chemical nature of the stone. The light band is broken up, and certain segments of the spectrum are absorbed while others are emanated, depending on the stone. The reflected bands of light are visible to the human eye as color. Because both color and gemstones emanate specific bands and vibrational levels of the spectrum, they are allied here in terms of therapeutic application.

Color can be utilized therapeutically in the following ways:

1) *Visualization*: the needed color is visualized as being inhaled and bathing body cells and tissues.

2) *Solarized Light*: the application of color-filtered sunlight to the affected area or chakra center. Both colored plastic gels and glass filters are used to adapt sunlight for this purpose.

3) *Solarized Water*: pure water is sun-exposed in the appropriate colored-glass container for one half hour and ingested as a vibrational medicine.[19]

Gemstones need to be cleansed and prepared for healing use. When you find or purchase stones for healing, size is not the important factor in their selection. Bigger stones do not necessarily make better or more potent healing stones. Choose stones of good color, quality and clarity, and avoid stones that have been cut, faceted or drilled. Stones that have been tumble-polished are fine to use (except in the case of quartz crystals, which must always be used in uncut, unpolished form).

When you have found a stone you wish to use in healing work, the first step is to bathe it in springwater or the water of a creek, river, stream or spring. Next, the stone is exposed to full sunlight for seven consecutive days, wrapping it away each evening during the exposure period. After the stones are washed and solarized, they are ready for healing work. They should not be worn as adornments or jewelry, but should be kept in a box or bag away from other items between healing uses.

---

[19]For descriptions of color treatment, see Alex Jones, *Seven Mansions of Color* (Marina del Rey, CA: DeVorss, 1977), pages 123–134; or Frank Don, *Color Your World* (Rochester, VT: Inner Traditions, 1987), pages 147–174.

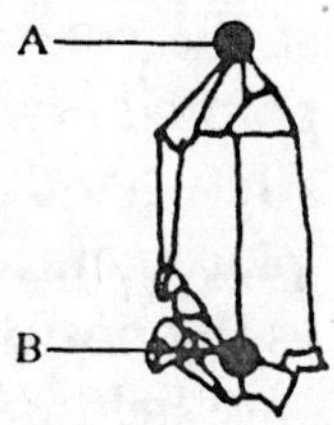

Figure 34. A typical quartz crystal. (A) indicates the terminal point; (B) indicates the matrix.

Each time a stone is used for a healing treatment, it must be cleared or neutralized in sea salt before using it again in another treatment. The stone is placed in a small container of dry sea salt for at least one half hour following each treatment use. In working with gemstones in healing, treatments should be spaced at least seven days apart.

The recipient of a gemstone treatment should always be positioned supine (lying on the back) with the head in a northerly or easterly direction. The therapy stone is placed in the subject's left hand. The healer then uses quartz crystals to amplify the vibrational intake of the therapy stone. Quartz crystal possesses a measurable piezoelectric pulse which amplifies polarity energy. Each crystal is also electrically directional, energy moving from the matrix toward the terminal (see figure 34). For this reason, both the crystals and the hands of the healer must be positioned properly to produce the polarity amplification.

In using the crystals to reinforce the vibrational intake of the therapy stone, the healer places one crystal against the sole of the subject's left foot with the terminal end of the crystal pointed toward the heel and holds the crystal in place with his or her right hand. The other crystal is placed against the sole of the subject's right foot with the terminal pointed toward the toes and held in place by the healer's left hand. Figure 35 illustrates the proper directional placement of the stones against the feet. Figure 36 shows the position of the subject and the healer. The crystals are held in place until an equalized temperature and a synchronized pulse are sensed in both feet, just as in balancing polarity therapy points. The balance of pulses signifies that the vibrational intake of the therapy stone is finished. After the treatment, all stones are placed in the sea salt to clear them before using them in another treatment.

It is important to note that while using the crystals to amplify the polarity-vibrational intake, the subject's expressed sensations will often be opposite to those of the healer. For example, after placing the therapy stone in the subject's left hand and positioning the crystals against the soles of the feet, the healer's first sensation may be a distinct feeling of coldness from the left foot,

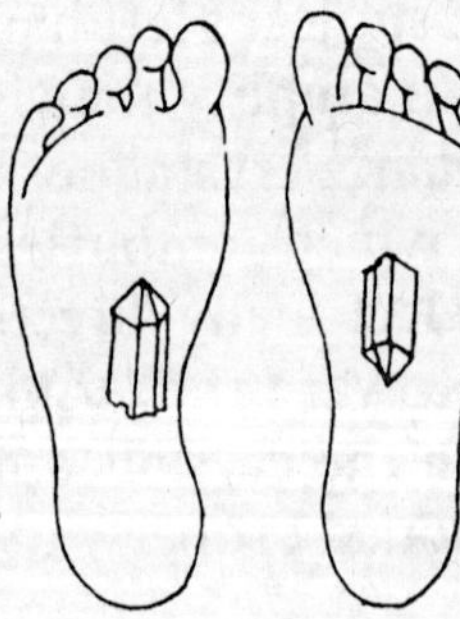

Figure 35. Placement of quartz crystals during a healing treatment.

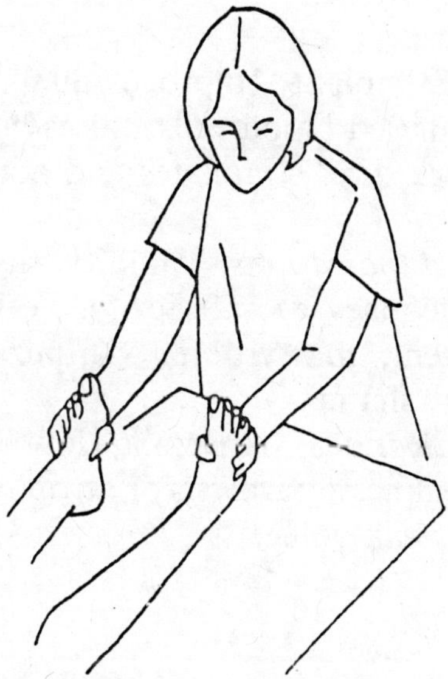

Figure 36. Position of healer and subject.

while the right foot feels hot. The subject will say the opposite: that the left foot feels warm while the right foot seems cold. This is because of the brain hemisphere crossover between the healer and the recipient. It is normal and not a sign that something is amiss in the treatment procedure.

Color and gemstone therapy is a treatment option available when imbalance (of chakra center, physical, or psychological polarities) has been detected. This section provides a color and gemstone guide and lists the chakra center resonated by each color and stone as well as the physical and psychological indications for which color or gem treatment may be used.

Red (436.7*)

Gemstone: Carnelian
Chakra: Sacral
Properties: Stimulant. Improves quality of blood and muscle, builds red blood cells, raises body temperature and blood pressure, stimulates and normalizes circulation.
Psychological indications: Timidity, shyness, feeling of failure, inadequacy or inferiority. Feelings of apathy, discouragement, martyrdom, victimization, low self-esteem, guilt, shame.
Physical indications: Anaemia, low blood pressure, muscular weakness, paralysis or atrophy, lethargy, poor circulation, weak voice.

Orange (473.6)

Gemstone: Amber
Chakra: Navel
Properties: Expectorant, antispasmodic, emmenagogue.
Psychological indications: Emotional and relationship stress, resentment, defensiveness, jealousy, envy, bitterness, possessiveness, fear of aging, loss, abandonment. Insecurity about image, appearance.
Physical indications: Respiratory disorders such as asthma, bronchitis, emphysema, cough; muscular spasm and cramping; menstrual difficulties and cramping; menopause, hormone imbalance.

---

*trillion vibrations per second.

Yellow (510.5)

Gemstone: Jade
Chakra: Solar Plexus
Properties: Nephritic, diuretic, digestive.
Psychological indications: Decision-making problems, poor concentration, preoccupation, inattention, memory lapses, informational overload, arguments (mental or verbal), obsessive thinking, prejudice, bias, mental rigidity.
Physical indications: Digestive tract disorders such as dyspepsia, diverticulosis, colitis, gastritis and the like; urinary tract disorders such as cystitis; sinus and allergy-like sensitivities; skin disorders; blood sugar imbalances and pancreatic disorders such as diabetes.

Green (584.3)

Gemstone: Turquoise
Chakra: Heart
Properties: Alternative, cardiac.
Psychological indications: Transition disorientation, disconnectedness.
Physical indications: To normalize heart action, cardiac arrhythmia or debility, palpitation, cholesterol deposits, high blood pressure, systemic toxicity, blood poisoning, tissue acidity or pH imbalance.

Blue (658.0)

Gemstone: Obsidian
Chakra: Throat
Properties: Diaphoretic, antiseptic.
Psychological indications: Hidden or suppressed grief, mourning, loss, emotional pain and scarring.
Physical indications: Fever, pain, infection, burns, wounds, injuries, bruises, swelling.

Indigo (694.9)

Gemstone: Aquamarine
Chakra: Brow
Properties: Nervine, demulcent, mild tranquilizer.
Psychological indications: Nervous agitation, hysteria, nightmares, delusions.
Physical indications: Addictions, nervous exhaustion, insomnia, restlessness; sensory impairments; stuttering; hearing or eyesight problems such as glaucoma, cataract, deafness, loss of physical balance.

Violet (731.8)

Gemstone: Amethyst
Chakra: Crown
Properties: Sedative, lymphatic, catabolic.
Psychological indications: Addictions, psychic negativity, feeling of possession, nightmares, hysteria, mental/emotional anguish.
Physical indications: Cravings, binges (food, alcohol, behavioral), hysteria, insomnia, neuritis, neuralgia, headaches, deposits in tissues or bloodstream, cysts, tumors, lymphatic debility or congestion.

HOMEOPATHIC REMEDY THERAPY

The term *homeopathy* is derived from Greek *homoios* (similar and *pathos* (suffering). The homeopathic school of medicine was founded nearly two hundred years ago by Dr. S. C. F. Hahnemann and based on the theory of treating "like with like." Hahnemann found that substances that elicit particular reactions in healthy individuals, when given in a material or toxic dose, could be utilized to alleviate similar conditions when given in microdoseages. Many of the breakthrough treatments of the last half of this century are based on this same theory—the theory of producing immunity through innoculation.

Homeopathy has always emphasized treatment of the individual as a totality, including beliefs, attitudes and emotions, as well as physical signs and symptoms. The focus in this type of treatment is the stimulation of the body's own defenses rather than suppression of symptoms. The homeopathic aim is reintegration, both physically and psychologically. Modern science is increasingly aware of the connection between stress and physical illness. Some researchers estimate that as much as ninety percent of physical disease is in fact psychologically based—caused, or at least facilitated, by tension, fear and anxiety. With proper homeopathic treatment, the damaged aspects of the personality begin to emerge. Because homeopathic treatment supports rather than suppresses trauma, it is particularly suited to psychological therapy, helping an individual to recognize and directly express his or her feelings. When emotional or psychological conflicts are found to underlie or reinstate chakra and meridian imbalances, the homeopathic remedies can be extremely valuable in resolving and releasing these conflicts.

Today there are hundreds of remedies for the treatment of both physical and psychological stresses. The remedies are officially recognized as medicines and listed in the Homeopathic Pharmacopeia of the United States.

The remedies are prepared and marketed in both liquid and tablet form. Depending on the form used, a single dose consists of one drop of liquid or one to three tablets. Remedies are available in potencies ranging from 3X to 30X. (Actually, higher potencies are manufactured, but it is not advised for the layperson or beginning practitioner to use potencies above 30X.) In general, the higher potencies (30X) act more quickly and at a deeper level than the lower (3X) ones.

Homeopathic remedies, whether tablet or liquid, should be deposited directly under the tongue and dissolved. Care should be taken not to contaminate the remedies while using them. If you are using the liquid form, avoid touching the dropper to tongue, mouth or fingers. Tablet doses should be poured into the bottle cap or onto a piece of paper. Do not return tablets that have been touched or handled back to the general supply bottle.

Response time and intensity varies with each individual. The remedies are self-adjusting, meaning that response occurs in harmony with individual need. A few guidelines concerning treatment with homeopathic remedies:[20]

1. The more severe the symptom-signs, the more frequently the doseage should be used. In mild situations, 3-4 doses per day are adequate. In more extreme situa-

[20]Stephen Cummings and Dana Ullman, *Everybody's Guide to Homeopathic Medicines* (Los Angeles: Jeremy Tarcher, 1984), pages 43-44.

tions, the dose may be repeated as frequently as every fifteen minutes.

2. Continue the treatment for at least three days. Allow time for the remedy to act. Sometimes there is a delayed response.

3. Use one remedy at a time. Although several remedies may be combined in one doseage, it is best to work with each remedy individually in order to avoid confusion or lack of clarity in recognizing and understanding the issues which each remedy stimulates.

It is important for the therapist to support the healthy and positive aspects of the client's personality during treatment and to maintain an open, non-judgmental attitude. Encouraging the client to keep a process journal while using the remedies, making short daily notes concerning emotions and sensations that surface during the treatment course, can also effectively enhance homeopathic therapy.

Table 4 on pages 138-145 groups the remedies according to predominant emotional issues and conflicts, and table 5 on pages 146-149 lists specific physical states. A brief psychological profile of each remedy will be found following the tables (and beginning) on pages 150-160. If chakra or meridian imbalance suggests the use of a homeopathic remedy, the remedy profile should be read carefully to determine whether it is a suitable treatment option.

You will find a listing of resource agencies and pharmacies for homeopathic remedies on page 190. In this book, we are listing homeopathic remedies by their common name first, followed by the Latin name in paretheses. Have both names handy when you order: some pharmacies will be geared toward using the Latin name; others will refer to the remedy by its common name.

Table 4 Psychological States

Symptom	Gemstone & Color							Homeopathic Remedy																	Aromatherapy							
	Carnelian/Red	Amber/Orange	Jade/Yellow	Turquoise/Green	Obsidian/Blue	Aquamarine/Indigo	Amethyst/Violet	Mullein/Nightshade	Wild Rose/Hellebore	Willow/Stavesacre	Holly/Chamomile	Mallow/Jasmine	St. Johnswort/Tree of Life	Rosemary/Club moss	Vervain/Thornapple	Skullcap/Wind Flower	Hawthorn/Ignatius	Comfrey/Leopard's-bane	Walnut/Club moss	Wild Oat/Windflower	Yarrow/Marking nut	Pine/Poison nut	Crabapple/Poison Ivy	Hyssop/Monkshood	Clove	Chamomile	Lavender	Jasmine	Eucalyptus	Sandalwood	Rose	Geranium
Absent-minded			●													●											●					
Addiction						●	●									●			●				●								●	
Aggression					●			●							●											●						
Agitation			●	●				●			●			●												●						
Anger		●			●			●		●	●															●					●	
Anxiety			●				●						●	●				●			●						●			●	●	●
Apathy	●								●																●							
Argumentativeness		●	●								●				●											●					●	
Arrogance						●		●							●																●	
Bitterness		●								●	●															●						
Broken heart				●	●												●	●										●				
Claustrophobia	●												●								●									●		●

Table 4 Psychological States (continued)

Symptom	Gemstone & Color							Homeopathic Remedy																	Aromatherapy							
	Carnelian/Red	Amber/Orange	Jade/Yellow	Turquoise/Green	Obsidian/Blue	Aquamarine/Indigo	Amethyst/Violet	Mullein/Nightshade	Wild Rose/Hellebore	Willow/Stavesacre	Holly/Chamomile	Mallow/Jasmine	St. Johnswort/Tree of Life	Rosemary/Club moss	Vervain/Thornapple	Skullcap/Wind Flower	Hawthorn/Ignatius	Comfrey/Leopard's-bane	Walnut/Club moss	Wild Oat/Windflower	Yarrow/Marking nut	Pine/Poison nut	Crabapple/Poison Ivy	Hyssop/Monkshood	Clove	Chamomile	Lavender	Jasmine	Eucalyptus	Sandalwood	Rose	Geranium
Complaining		●								●	●															●						
Compulsiveness		●											●								●									●		
Confusion			●											●		●											●					
Criticalness			●					●		●	●				●											●					●	
Cynicism	●	●								●	●															●					●	
Day dreaming			●						●					●		●									●							
Defensiveness		●								●	●				●											●						
Depression	●				●				●	●			●				●				●				●			●		●		●
Despair	●				●								●				●				●							●		●		●
Discouraged	●								●	●							●	●												●		●
Disoriented				●													●							●								●
Doubt	●											●				●	●											●				

Table 4 Psychological States (continued)	Gemstone & Color							Homeopathic Remedy																	Aromatherapy							
Symptom	Carnelian/Red	Amber/Orange	Jade/Yellow	Turquoise/Green	Obsidian/Blue	Aquamarine/Indigo	Amethyst/Violet	Mullein/Nightshade	Wild Rose/Hellebore	Willow/Stavesacre	Holly/Chamomile	Mallow/Jasmine	St. Johnswort/Tree of Life	Rosemary/Club moss	Vervain/Thornapple	Skullcap/Wind Flower	Hawthorn/Ignatius	Comfrey/Leopard's-bane	Walnut/Club moss	Wild Oat/Windflower	Yarrow/Marking nut	Pine/Poison nut	Crabapple/Poison Ivy	Hyssop/Monkshood	Clove	Chamomile	Lavender	Jasmine	Eucalyptus	Sandalwood	Rose	Geranium
Envy		●									●															●						
Fear, general	●								●				●								●			●						●		●
—of loss		●									●	●	●				●													●		●
—of failure	●								●	●			●																	●		
—of death	●												●								●			●						●		●
—of aging		●										●	●															●		●		
—of commitment			●										●			●				●										●		
—of rejection	●	●								●	●	●	●																	●		
—of abandonment		●									●	●	●															●		●		
Frustration	●							●		●																●						
Grief	●				●												●	●						●				●				●

Table 4 Psychological States (continued)

	Gemstone & Color							Homeopathic Remedy																	Aromatherapy							
Symptom	Carnelian/Red	Amber/Orange	Jade/Yellow	Turquoise/Green	Obsidian/Blue	Aquamarine/Indigo	Amethyst/Violet	Mullein/Nightshade	Wild Rose/Hellebore	Willow/Stavesacre	Holly/Chamomile	Mallow/Jasmine	St. Johnswort/Tree of Life	Rosemary/Club moss	Vervain/Thornapple	Skullcap/Wind Flower	Hawthorn/Ignatius	Comfrey/Leopard's-bane	Walnut/Club moss	Wild Oat/Windflower	Yarrow/Marking nut	Pine/Poison nut	Crabapple/Poison Ivy	Hyssop/Monkshood	Clove	Chamomile	Lavender	Jasmine	Eucalyptus	Sandalwood	Rose	Geranium
Guilt	•												•									•	•					•			•	
Hallucination			•			•	•						•								•									•		•
Hatred		•									•															•						
Hopelessness	•			•	•								•				•				•									•		•
Hostility		•								•	•															•						
Hyperactivity				•															•	•							•					
Hysteria	•						•						•								•			•						•		•
Identity crisis	•																		•	•					•							
Impatience			•					•							•											•	•					
Impulsiveness			•		•			•																			•					
Indecisiveness			•													•											•					
Indifference	•								•								•								•							

Table 4 Psychological States (continued)	Gemstone & Color							Homeopathic Remedy																	Aromatherapy							
Symptom	Carnelian/Red	Amber/Orange	Jade/Yellow	Turquoise/Green	Obsidian/Blue	Aquamarine/Indigo	Amethyst/Violet	Mullein/Nightshade	Wild Rose/Hellebore	Willow/Stavesacre	Holly/Chamomile	Mallow/Jasmine	St. Johnswort/Tree of Life	Rosemary/Club moss	Vervain/Thornapple	Skullcap/Wind Flower	Hawthorn/Ignatius	Comfrey/Leopard's-bane	Walnut/Club moss	Wild Oat/Windflower	Yarrow/Marking nut	Pine/Poison nut	Crabapple/Poison Ivy	Hyssop/Monkshood	Clove	Chamomile	Lavender	Jasmine	Eucalyptus	Sandalwood	Rose	Geranium
Inferiority	•								•			•	•										•		•							
Intolerance			•					•							•											•	•					
Irrationality				•																				•				•				•
Irritability		•						•			•															•						
Jealousy		•									•															•						
Lethargy	•								•								•								•							
Loneliness		•						•		•		•	•				•											•				
Loss of faith	•				•								•				•				•							•				
Martyrdom	•								•								•								•							
Memory loss			•											•	•									•			•					
Mood swings				•														•									•					

Table 4 Psychological States (continued)

Symptom	Gemstone & Color							Homeopathic Remedy																	Aromatherapy							
	Carnelian/Red	Amber/Orange	Jade/Yellow	Turquoise/Green	Obsidian/Blue	Aquamarine/Indigo	Amethyst/Violet	Mullein/Nightshade	Wild Rose/Hellebore	Willow/Stavesacre	Holly/Chamomile	Mallow/Jasmine	St. Johnswort/Tree of Life	Rosemary/Club moss	Vervain/Thornapple	Skullcap/Wind Flower	Hawthorn/Ignatius	Comfrey/Leopard's-bane	Walnut/Club moss	Wild Oat/Windflower	Yarrow/Marking nut	Pine/Poison nut	Crabapple/Poison Ivy	Hyssop/Monkshood	Clove	Chamomile	Lavender	Jasmine	Eucalyptus	Sandalwood	Rose	Geranium
Narrow minded			•					•							•												•					
Neglect, feeling of		•								•	•															•		•				
Nightmares		•					•						•								•			•						•		•
Obsession		•	•				•						•								•						•			•		•
Panic	•	•		•									•					•			•			•						•		
Paranoia			•											•							•						•			•		•
Persecution		•								•	•															•						
Phobia		•	•				•						•	•							•						•			•		•
Poor concentration			•													•											•					
Poor self image	•								•														•		•			•				
Possessiveness		•									•															•						

Table 4 Psychological States (continued)	Gemstone & Color							Homeopathic Remedy																	Aromatherapy							
Symptom	Carnelian/Red	Amber/Orange	Jade/Yellow	Turquoise/Green	Obsidian/Blue	Aquamarine/Indigo	Amethyst/Violet	Mullein/Nightshade	Wild Rose/Hellebore	Willow/Stavesacre	Holly/Chamoinile	Mallow/Jasmine	St. Johnswort/Tree of Life	Rosemary/Club moss	Vervain/Thornapple	Skullcap/Wind Flower	Hawthorn/Ignatius	Comfrey/Leopard's-bane	Walnut/Club moss	Wild Oat/Windflower	Yarrow/Marking nut	Pine/Poison nut	Crabapple/Poison Ivy	Hyssop/Monkshood	Clove	Chamomile	Lavender	Jasmine	Eucalyptus	Sandalwood	Rose	Geranium
Possession			●				●						●								●						●			●		●
Prejudice			●					●							●											●	●					
Preoccupation			●											●		●											●					
Procrastination			●													●											●					
Resentment		●								●	●															●					●	
Revenge		●									●															●						
Rigidity			●												●												●					
Self-absorption	●							●		●	●			●												●	●					
Self-consciousness	●											●											●					●				
Self-doubt			●													●																
Self-pity	●			●						●																		●				

Table 4 Psychological States (continued)

Symptom	Gemstone & Color							Homeopathic Remedy																	Aromatherapy							
	Carnelian/Red	Amber/Orange	Jade/Yellow	Turquoise/Green	Obsidian/Blue	Aquamarine/Indigo	Amethyst/Violet	Mullein/Nightshade	Wild Rose/Hellebore	Willow/Stavesacre	Holly/Chamomile	Mallow/Jasmine	St. Johnswort/Tree of Life	Rosemary/Club moss	Vervain/Thornapple	Skullcap/Wind Flower	Hawthorn/Ignatius	Comfrey/Leopard's-bane	Walnut/Club moss	Wild Oat/Windflower	Yarrow/Marking nut	Pine/Poison nut	Crabapple/Poison Ivy	Hyssop/Monkshood	Clove	Chamomile	Lavender	Jasmine	Eucalyptus	Sandalwood	Rose	Geranium
Self Reproach			●													●						●	●									
Self Righteousness			●												●												●					
Shame	●																					●	●						●			
Shyness	●								●			●											●					●				
Shock/trauma	●				●								●											●						●		
Superiority			●												●											●	●					
Suspicion		●									●															●	●					
Uncertainty	●	●	●													●			●	●												
Victimization	●								●														●		●				●			
Worry			●											●		●		●									●					
Withdrawal	●								●	●							●								●							

Table 5 Physical States

Symptom	Gemstone & Color							Min/Vitamin							Aromatherapy Oil											Chakra						
	Carnelian/Red	Amber/Orange	Jade/Yellow	Turquoise/Green	Obsidian/Blue	Aquamarine/Indigo	Amethyst/Violet	Iron/E	Calcium/B Comp	Silicon/A	Potass/C	Iodine/K	Magnes/B Comp	Lithium/D	Clove	Geranium	Peppermint	Lavender	Jasmine	Eucalyptus	Sandalwood	Rose	Basil	Juniper	Cedarwood	Sacral	Navel	Solar Plexus	Heart	Throat	Brow	Crown
Acidosis				●							●													●					●			
Addiction						●	●						●	●								●									●	●
Anaemia	●							●							●								●			●						
Arthritis		●		●					●		●													●			●		●			
Asthma		●							●											●	●				●		●					
Bladder condition			●							●	●										●			●				●				
Blood poisoning				●							●													●					●			
Blood sugar			●							●									●									●				
Bronchial condition		●							●											●	●				●		●					
Burns					●			●	●	●	●	●				●		●			●	●			●					●		
Cholesterol level				●				●			●													●					●			

Table 5 Physical States (continued)

Symptom	Gemstone & Color							Min/Vitamin							Aromatherapy Oil											Chakra						
	Carnelian/Red	Amber/Orange	Jade/Yellow	Turquoise/Green	Obsidian/Blue	Aquamarine/Indigo	Amethyst/Violet	Iron/E	Calcium/B Comp	Silicon/A	Potass/C	Iodine/K	Magnes/B Comp	Lithium/D	Clove	Geranium	Peppermint	Lavender	Jasmine	Eucalyptus	Sandalwood	Rose	Basil	Juniper	Cedarwood	Sacral	Navel	Solar Plexus	Heart	Throat	Brow	Crown
Cold, flu					●						●						●			●				●						●		
Digestive condition			●					●		●	●				●		●						●					●				
Eczema			●					●		●	●					●		●			●	●			●			●				
Epilepsy		●							●								●										●					
Eyes						●	●	●	●	●	●		●			●						●									●	
Exhaustion	●							●	●	●	●				●								●			●						
Fever					●						●						●			●										●		
General detoxification				●							●							●						●					●			
Headache					●								●		●		●	●					●			●				●		
Hearing loss						●	●															●			●						●	
Heart conditions				●				●			●						●	●	●					●					●			

Table 5 Physical States (continued)

Symptom	Gemstone & Color							Min/Vitamin							Aromatherapy Oil											Chakra						
	Carnelian/Red	Amber/Orange	Jade/Yellow	Turquoise/Green	Obsidian/Blue	Aquamarine/Indigo	Amethyst/Violet	Iron/E	Calcium/B Comp	Silicon/A	Potass/C	Iodine/K	Magnes/B Comp	Lithium/D	Clove	Geranium	Peppermint	Lavender	Jasmine	Eucalyptus	Sandalwood	Rose	Basil	Juniper	Cedarwood	Sacral	Navel	Solar Plexus	Heart	Throat	Brow	Crown
Herpes					●											●	●			●		●								●		
Hormone imbalance		●						●	●	●	●					●			●								●					
Hypertension or hypotension				●				●			●						●	●	●					●					●			
Immune deficiency					●		●	●	●	●	●	●	●	●		●				●		●	●			●				●		●
Infection					●			●	●	●	●	●	●	●				●		●				●						●		
Insomnia			●				●	●	●	●			●	●		●	●	●			●							●				●
Liver condition		●							●		●										●			●			●					
Lung condition		●						●	●	●	●									●	●				●		●					
Lymphatic congestion	●						●	●	●	●	●	●	●		●							●	●	●		●				●		●
Menopause	●	●						●	●	●	●	●	●	●		●			●							●	●					
Menses difficulties		●						●	●				●			●			●								●					

Table 5 Physical States (continued)

Symptom	Gemstone & Color							Min/Vitamin							Aromatherapy Oil											Chakra						
	Carnelian/Red	Amber/Orange	Jade/Yellow	Turquoise/Green	Obsidian/Blue	Aquamarine/Indigo	Amethyst/Violet	Iron/E	Calcium/B Comp	Silicon/A	Potass/C	Iodine/K	Magnes/B Comp	Lithium/D	Clove	Geranium	Peppermint	Lavender	Jasmine	Eucalyptus	Sandalwood	Rose	Basil	Juniper	Cedarwood	Sacral	Navel	Solar Plexus	Heart	Throat	Brow	Crown
Muscle injury					•			•	•	•	•						•	•												•		
Neuritis							•		•					•		•	•				•											•
Overweight	•						•								•					•			•			•						•
Respiratory problems		•						•	•	•	•									•	•				•		•					
Sinus			•						•	•	•		•				•	•						•				•				
Skin conditions			•					•		•	•					•		•				•			•			•				
Stuttering						•	•						•	•						•				•							•	
Throat problems					•			•		•	•							•		•	•				•					•		
Urinary tract cond.			•					•		•	•										•			•				•				
Viral infections					•						•						•	•		•	•			•						•		
Wounds					•			•		•	•					•		•	•		•	•			•					•		

Shame and Guilt

Crabapple (Malus coronaria)

The crabapple remedy is useful for feelings of contamination, shame and poor self-image. It is especially helpful for those who have been victimized or abused, and helps to release traces of regret and disgust. This remedy assists in the cleansing and release of toxins on all levels—physical, mental and emotional. It is also helpful in releasing bad habits or guilty and unpleasant memories.

Poison Ivy (Rhus toxicodendron)

Like crabapple, the poison ivy remedy is valuable in assisting in cleansing and detoxification programs and in releasing memories of self-disgust and shame. It is also of benefit to those who are ashamed or self-conscious of their appearance and especially when physical scars, deformities or blemishes have damaged self-image and confidence.

Grief

St. Ignatius Bean (Ignatia)

The Ignatius remedy is useful in situations of unresolved grief, when the mourning process has been suppressed or interrupted. There is often the constant feeling of a lump in the throat. The Ignatius type is reluctant to share their pain and suffering, they dread making a scene and fear the loss of emotional control.

Hawthorn (Crataegus oxycantha)

Hawthorn remedy is for the broken-hearted, those who suffer from grief, loss and separation and feelings of emptiness due to trauma. Hawthorn is for those who feel they have lost or sacrificed so much that they can no longer feel anything. It brings comfort and release from feelings of deadness and numbness.

See also *White Hellebore*.

Shock and Trauma

Hyssop (Hyssopus officinale)
The hyssop remedy functions like a stabilizer following periods of trauma. The hyssop type usually manifests a stunned, speechless reaction to sudden or unexpected shocks and events. It is the remedy for disorientation, following crisis or the receiving of sad or serious news.

Monkshood (Aconitum napellus)
The monkshood remedy is useful in cases of terror, trauma and accident. The monkshood type usually reacts to shock with restlessness, hysteria, fidgeting, talking to themselves or even wandering about with little awareness of where they are or what they are doing. Monkshood should be used following any episode of fright, shock or accident.

Comfrey (Symphytum officinale)
Comfrey is the remedy for the wracked, for those who feel they have been through one thing after another and have suffered both physically and emotionally. It is for those who feel weary to the core. Often the physical vitality is sapped and the adrenals are weakened. Reserve strength is lost. Comfrey gives the courage to

face what looks like the impossible and carry on. It helps one to roll with the punches.

Leopard's-bane (Arnica)
The Leopard's-bane type feels "beat up," bruised and damaged. The entire body aches after episodes of grief, remorse or sudden loss. Leopard's-bane is the remedy of choice whenever trauma has resulted in actual physical injury, no matter how minor. It is also especially useful in releasing fears and tensions which are the emotional aftermath of long ago incidents of injury, violence or abuse.

Apathy and Withdrawal

Rose (Rosea)
The rose type is apathetic, "drifts," resigned to accept all without making any attempt to change. They "throw in the towel" and give up without a fight. They may feel used or victimized, but unable or unwilling to do anything about it. They are martyrs, and often feel timid, inferior or subservient. The rose remedy helps people to learn to speak out and stand up for what is important to them. It helps to develop more ambition, direction and initiative.

White Hellebore (Veratrum album)
Hellebore should be considered whenever profound apathy and withdrawal are present. The hellebore type seems closed and indifferent, refuses to talk or interact. They feel defeated by fate and events, and react with silent withdrawal. The hellebore type believes that all is lost and hopeless and does not feel that recovery or improvement are possible. Hellebore helps to re-establish faith and optimism.

Fear and Phobia

St. Johnswort (Hypericum perforatum)
The St. Johnswort type is anxious and apprehensive, sometimes for no known or apparent reason. They may have fear of hunger, poverty, the dark, and so on. This remedy helps to release fears from both known and unknown causes. Phobias and compulsions, from childhood or even unidentified sources, can be released through the use of this remedy. It is very useful in nightmare. It brings increased ease to mind and body, acts as a mild tranquilizer.

Tree of Life (Thuja occidentalis)
The tree of life type seems stubborn and obsessional about their fears, they refuse to be argued or reasoned out of their anxieties. They are often convinced that a tumor or foreign substance in the brain or body is the cause of all their problems. They are emotionally hypersensitive and swing between enthusiasm and tearful depression. Their fears are physically exhausting, causing insomnia and restless sleep. Tree of life acts as a stabilizer and tranquilizer.

Yarrow (Achillea millifolium)
Yarrow remedy helps to release negative thought-forms and feelings of psychic vulnerablity or even possession. It strengthens and protects the auric shield and is very helpful in nervous hysteria, nerve sensitivity, insomnia and disorientation.

Marking Nut (Anacardium)
The marking nut type fears loss of control, they are afraid they may do something awful or unforgiveable. They feel separated, as though living in a dream. The

sensory world seems distant and unreal. They often report feeling "split," as though living in two worlds or accompanied by another, invisible self. They may hear voices or experience visual hallucinations. The marking nut remedy helps to stabilize and ground the personality in present surroundings.

Defensiveness, Anger and Jealousy

Willow (Salix)
Willow remedy helps release feelings of resentment, bitterness and self-pity. The willow type may suffer from a persecution complex, feeling that the world always hands them the short straw. It is the remedy for those who feel that their situation is somehow unjust or unfair. They may withdraw from others to avoid further disillusionment or rejection, and develop a cynical attitude as a defense mechanism. They may "sulk" in corners, hoping someone will notice their loneliness and unhappiness.

Chamomile (Chamomilla)
Chamomile is the remedy of choice whenever there is a tendency toward unreasonable irritability and complaining. Because of deep-seated insecurity, the chamomile type can be extremely demanding in their need for constant attention and affection. Unfortunately, they often use nagging or whining as a means of obtaining the attention they crave. They may even go to the extremes of tantrums or dramatic emotional displays. Chamomile helps to calm the emotions and develop trust and gentleness.

Holly (Ilex aquifolium)

The holly type is suspicious and wary in relationships. They maintain a low-grade, unconscious surliness. Deep down inside they are waiting to be rejected or abandoned, because they do not truly believe they deserve to be loved. They are defensive and frequently involved in hostilities and misunderstandings with others. Privately, they may feel envious or jealous of others, or feel they are not appreciated or understood. The holly remedy helps release feelings of hostility and bitterness and develop attitudes of charity and peacefulness. Holly helps in learning to accept love.

Nightshade (Belladonna)

Nightshade is the remedy to consider when dealing with anger and the "hair-trigger" personality. The mood of the nightshade type can change suddenly and dramatically. They can be meek as a lamb one minute and mad as a hornet the next. They can be verbally abusive and even violent in the heat of an argument. One of the characteristics of the nightshade type is the tendency toward redness and facial flushing when emotionally upset. The nightshade remedy releases anger and helps to balance mood swings.

Mullein (Verbascum thapsus)

The mullein type is easily irritated, impatient and perfectionistic. They do everything quickly and efficiently. They move speedily, finish other people's sentences for them, and are sometimes accident-prone because of their haste and impetuosity. They pressure both themselves and others and often work alone in order to avoid the frustration and delays of slower co-workers. The result is that they often feel isolated and unappreciated. Mullein remedy helps people to learn to take things one at a time, and to develop a more relaxed and flexible energy flow.

Stavesacre (Staphysagria)

Stavesacre can be well used whenever there is a tendency to retain hurt and anger with the desire for revenge. The stavesacre type may act casually amiable following an insult or slight to their pride, but they can remember and harbor resentment for years. This remedy facilitates the ability to "forgive and forget."

Vervain (Verbena hastata)

The vervain type is extremist, possessing strong convictions and opinions. They are strongly self-reliant and self-willed. They can be very critical, even tyrannical, in imposing their ideas and viewpoints on others. They are highstrung and often push the body to the limits of endurance. Vervain remedy helps to develop more open-mindedness, empathy and tolerance. It brings more balance to the thinking and manner of communicating.

Thornapple (Stramonium)

Like vervain, the thornapple remedy is used to soften and balance mental and verbal extremes. The thornapple type tends to be more obsessional and delusional in their thinking than the vervain type. They are propagandizers, soap-boxers, the "fire and brimstone" preachers, attempting through emotional force and verbal barrage to coerce others and reduce any opposition to their own rigid viewpoints. Thornapple remedy helps to broaden the viewpoint, develop more forbearance, cooperation and respect for others' lifestyles.

Uncertainty and Self-Consciousness

Mallow (Malva sylvestris)
The mallow type is uncertain about their physical appearance, attractiveness and image. They fear aging and may be compulsive about fashion, fads, and cosmetics in an effort to assuage their inner fears. Mallow remedy helps these people to develop more certainty about self-worth and desirability. It helps release fears of aging and fosters self-acceptance and self-appreciation.

Yellow Jasmine (Gelsemium)
Jasmine is the remedy of choice whenever there is an overwhelming attack of stage fright or panic. The jasmine type is always projecting into the future and imagining all sorts of disasters and failures. Outwardly they may appear calm and cheerful, but inside they are undone, victims of "butterflies in the stomach." Jasmine is an excellent remedy to use prior to public appearances, examinations or other events which cause anxiety over what *might* happen.

Skullcap (Skulletaria lateriflora)
The skullcap type talks a lot and is the "hail fellow, well met," gregarious, seeking approval and advice for every plan and idea. They often have trouble discerning their priorities and values, and continually waver between decisions. They are information addicts, and are often labeled procrastinators because of their overreliance on information before being able to act on their decisions. They are often addictive or repeater personalities, leaning on people, advice or substances to help them solve their problems. The skullcap remedy strengthens, quiets

and deepens the mind and helps build confidence in inner guidance and judgment.

Walnut (Juglans regia)
Walnut remedy is for those who are in the midst of transition. Walnut helps a person to break free of old behaviors and habits. This remedy helps to bear the severance from familiar circumstances. Walnut remedy is appropriate for any type of transition in life, to assist in moving into the new and unknown.

Windflower (Pulsatilla)
Windflower is the remedy of choice in situations of indecision. It is usually agonizing for the windflower type to make a commitment. They are insecure, easily led and influenced by others, and very vulnerable to outside advice and circumstances. The windflower personality is often preoccupied with partners and relationships as a means of unconsciously building their own self-worth. The windflower remedy helps develop firm resolution, confidence, and personal values.

Oat (Avena sativa)
The oat type is often frustrated by their lack of ability to bring ideas to fruition. They are often quite talented and very resourceful, but they seem to lack focus or the ability to prioritize. They scatter energies among too many projects or expressions. Oat remedy helps to focus, center and develop skills and talents. It helps to develop self-discipline and initiative and is a good remedy to use during periods of career or creative uncertainty.

Club Moss (Lycopodium)
Club moss remedy is useful whenever there is evidence of weakened memory and poor concentration. The moss type often loses their train of thought, forgets names and so on. They are great idea people, but sometimes use their intellectual flights as a means of escape or to avoid involvement. They are "armchair philosophers." The moss remedy helps to steady the mind and ground the mental energies, it helps these people come out of the clouds.

Tension and Anxiety

Pine (Pinus sylvestris)
Pine is the remedy for those who experience tension due to their inability to rectify or reclaim the past. They continually blame or fault themselves, and are never content or satisfied with their efforts. They always feel they could have done better. They are secretly self-reproachful, overly-conscientious and dissatisifed. Pine remedy helps to learn to forgive self and release the past.

Rosemary (Rosmarinus officinale)
The rosemary type has a highly active and alert mind, often cluttered with opposing views and circling thoughts that run on like broken records. Their thoughts seem obsessive and persistent and drive out mental peace and clarity. The rosemary type may seem preoccupied, forgetful, or inattentive because of their over-active and distracting thoughts. The rosemary remedy helps to develop attention and clarity. It helps cleanse the mind of unnecessary clutter, agitation and congestion.

Poison Nut (Nux vomica)
Poison nut is the remedy of choice for situations of mental strain, overwork and nervous tension. The poison nut types are worrywarts, they over-focus and over-magnify minor matters and fret themselves to exhaustion. They are prone to insomnia, perfectionistic, and rarely leave their work behind at the end of the day. Their anxious thoughts seem to run away with them and sap vitality. The poison nut remedy assists in learning to relax, release mental tension and develop detachment and perspective.

HEALING THE HEALER

Any type of counseling or therapy work can be extremely demanding, even draining at times. When you are working with body polarity and vibrational therapy, you are working with extremely subtle energy states. Because these forms of healing involve the manipulation of such subtle and potent energies, the effects on your own body can be easily overlooked or difficult to assess. Vibrational therapists need to exercise special care in maintaining and regenerating themselves.

This book has concerned itself with energy blockages and accumulations, and subtle healing methods for resolving imbalances. As therapists, we must remember that we are also (and always) human beings, each with our own set of conflicts and "hang-ups."

Vibrational therapists, consciously or otherwise, are consistently utilizing the higher glandular centers in the body in order to do their work. This places a tremendous vibrational strain on the physical body and creates the distinct possibility of overload and degeneration, depending on the therapist's own weak spots. Therapists who use such energies must learn to attune and adjust the physical body, and especially the nervous system, to higher octave vibrational levels in order to avoid exhaustion and breakdown. If the higher glandular centers become misaligned, for whatever reason, these therapists will be forced to draw on the lower centers to continue working. This leads to further weakening and eventual depletion of both the physiological and psychological structures. Often therapists may feel that their work is somehow invalidated or that they are "failing" in some way if they must admit the need for rest and recuperation. Concepts about self-importance and personal power may actually be obstructing effective functioning as a therapist (and as a human being). It takes courage to admit that you are "only" human.

Signs and symptoms that may be indicating the need for rest and realignment include:

Sudden weight changes: gaining may signify the body's attempt to insulate and shield itself; losses indicate depletion and draining.

Nervous system stress: mood swings; significant shifts in sleep or dream patterns, such as insomnia or extreme lethargy; muscular tensions, headaches, breathing irregularities or difficulties.

Disruption of the menstrual cycle may be indicative of excessive physical strain or depletion.

To strengthen and maintain ourselves as vibrational therapists, we need to be conscious of diet—getting plenty of daily fluids, adequate protein, foods and vitamins which nourish the nervous system such as

B complex and C vitamins and foods, magnesium, calcium, trace minerals and lecithin. We need regular physical exercise to tone the lymphatic and circulatory structures and to help ground us and discharge static accumulations. Breathing and meditation exercises before and after healing sessions help to clear the energies and prevent static accumulations. Last, but not least, we should try to remember to use the very tools we use to help heal others—to heal ourselves. The old adage, "The cobbler's children have no shoes," is just as appropriate to therapists and counselors. Often, the last thing that occurs to us as therapists is to apply some of the same healing methods and understandings we use everyday to help others, to heal ourselves. Sometimes someone else actually has to point out to us that we could use a little of "our own medicine." As therapists we should be humble and brave enough to seek the assistance of a colleague when and if we need it.

CHAPTER FIVE

Review

Now that you've become familiar with chakras, meridians, balancing points and forms of treatment therapy, let's review the treatment outline for chakra center assessment and balancing. Figure 37 on page 164 will help you review the balancing points.

Position the individual to be assessed or balanced supine (lying on the back), with the head in a northerly or easterly direction.

Use the pendulum to assess the energy vortex at each center. If a center imbalance is detected you should:

- Wind the center & balance the electromagnetic pulse points that readjust the center energies.
- Choose one of the essential oils that stimulates the center and apply it to the center anointing point.
- Examine the four meridians networking to/from the center. If you locate an affected meridian:

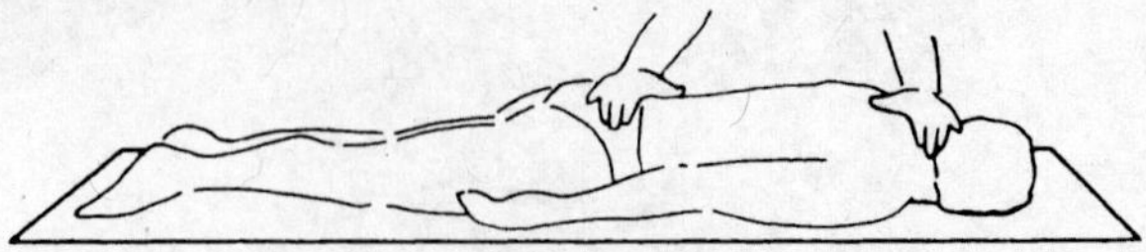

A. Sacral chakra

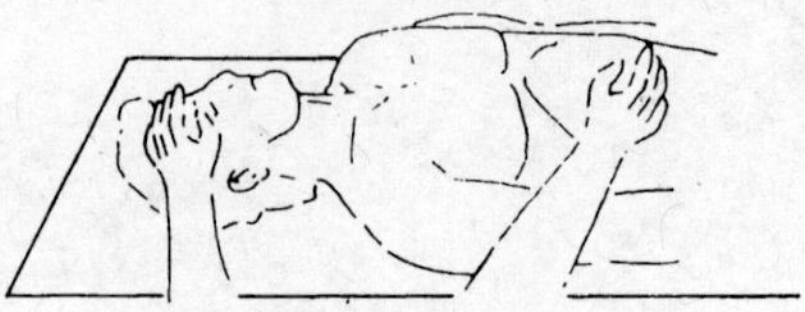

B. Navel chakra

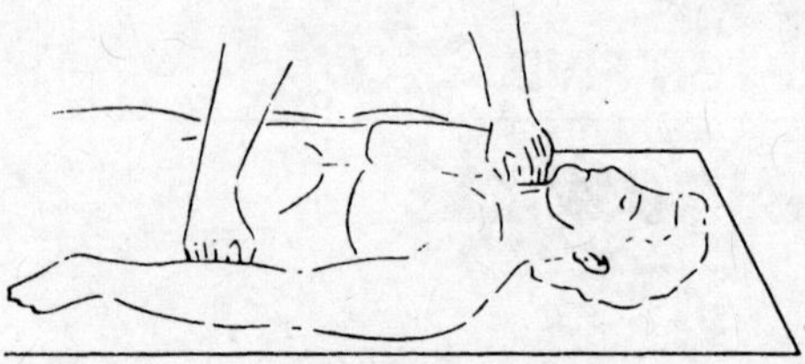

C. Solar Plexus chakra

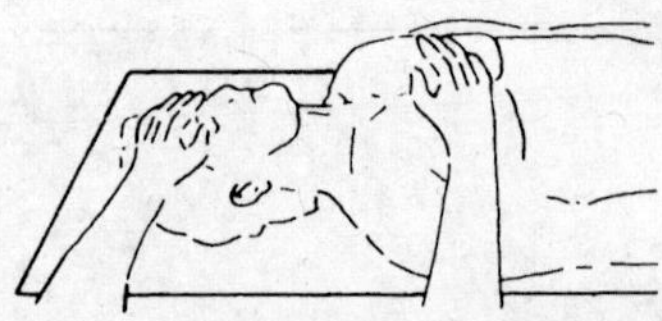

D. Heart chakra

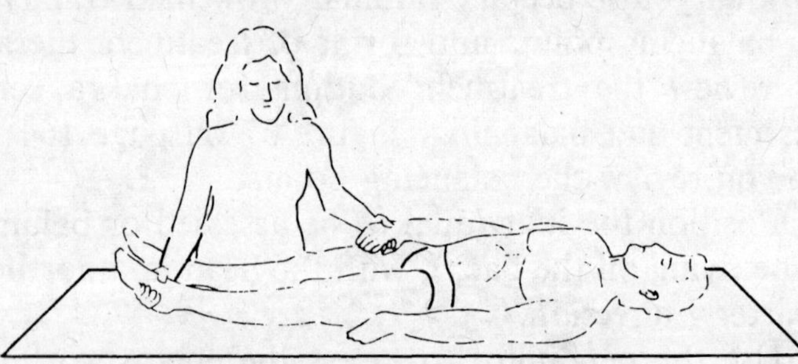

E. Throat chakra

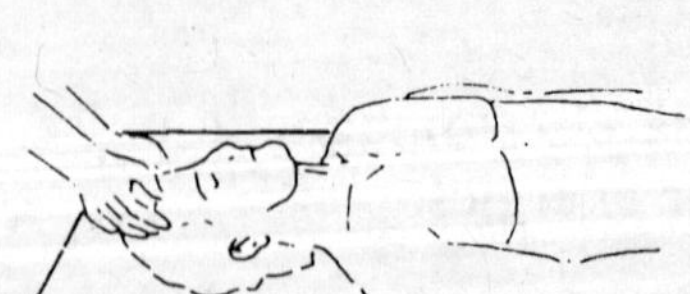

F. Brow chakra

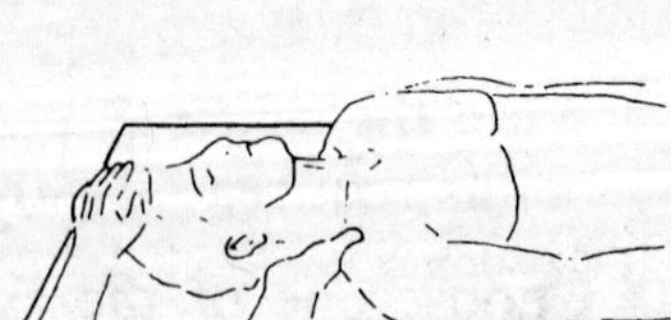

G. Crown chakra

Figure 37. Chakra balancing points.

1) Readjust the meridian energies;

2) Apply appropriate myotherapy to affected muscles;

3) Identify the psycho-social conflict that imbalances the meridian and reinstates energy disturbance: a) Select a homeopathic remedy that will assist in releasing identified stress; b) develop counseling interactions appropriate to identified conflict.

4) Utilize the vibrational treatments (color and gemstone) that will facilitate release of the disturbed center's residues and impressions.

CHAPTER SIX

Case Notes

In developing and working with vibrational therapy, I have witnessed some remarkable incidents. In presenting these case notes, I hope to demonstrate how some of the concepts and methods introduced in this book can be integrated into counseling and healing practice. Although there are startling aspects to each of these cases, they were not chosen because of their unusual quality or uniqueness. In fact, they are typical, in my opinion and experience, of the sorts of interactions which occur in vibrational treatment.

There are several things in vibrational treatment which consistently strike me as significant:

First, the treatment seems to stimulate, *within a matter of minutes*, the discovery or release of incidents or conflicts which have been deeply buried and suppressed beneath conscious awareness. Generally, it may require many hours or even months of careful counseling to uncover this type of conflict.

Secondly, the treatment seems to enhance patients' own holistic or right brain awareness. They often make revealing and fascinating connections between the physical and psychological aspects of their problem, between the symbolic and the concrete. They do this on their own, with no prompting from me. I am as surprised and intrigued by their insights as they seem to be.

And thirdly (and this is the most difficult to articulate), the treatment seems to have the quality of, or to unfold within, a different sort of time framework than the one we are normally, consciously aware of. There is a dream-like sense of time during the treatment sessions, a sense of time out of time, of some displacement from the ordinary conscious context and sensation of time.

CASE 1

Julie M. first came to me for massage therapy which we both hoped would correct, or at least improve, a set of minor physical problems. She was thirty-two years old, married, independently employed in challenging and creative work. She was successful, relatively happy and optimistic about her future. After three months of weekly sessions, we had made marked progress in terms of our original objectives. She was pleased with the results of our sessions and said that she now looked forward to the treatments, not just as a part of her health care program, but also because of the relaxing and personal nature of the work. I was as pleased as Julie, but as we had made progress together, I had come to notice another situation which had, at first, been overlooked by our attention to other, more pressing matters. The problem was that the quadriceps muscles on the front of the thighs were so consistently tense and tightened that no matter how much I worked, what techniques I used, or how many sessions we had, these muscles never relaxed. I was curious about this, and in our thirteenth session I called it to Julie's attention. I felt, if she was willing, that we should try to make some progress on this tension, to take another step further now that our original objectives in treatment had been reached. Julie was a very pragmatic, no-nonsense type and I was a bit hesitant to suggest the vibrational therapies, thinking she might find them "weird" or unscientific. But after discussing the situation and agreeing that we had tried a varicty of physical therapies to try to release the muscle stress, she was curious to see what a more subtle, non-manipulative method might achieve.

The extreme tension of the quadriceps muscle indicated a disturbance of the small intestine meridian circuit networking to and from the sacral chakra center. In assessing Julie's chakra centers, I found, not surprisingly, the sacral center to be disturbed as well. I readjusted the sacral center energies using the electromagnetic pulse points (skull base and sacrum), anointed the base of the brain with neroli oil, and placed a small piece of carnelian (stone resonant to the sacral chakra) in Julie's left hand. Next, I placed the quartz crystals against the soles of her feet to amplify the vibrational effect of the carnelian. I then quietly held the crystals in place, awaiting the balancing of the foot pulses. The crystals had been in place against her feet for about three minutes, when Julie suddenly sat bolt upright on the table and said "I tried to run! I tried to run!" She had a sleepy, slightly bewildered, faraway look like someone who had just awakened from a bad dream. "Tried to run?" I asked. She blinked a few times, seemingly surprised to find herself there on the massage table. She seemed confused and embarrassed. "Tried to run?" I asked her again. She then haltingly and with obvious deep shame and embarrassment, told me that she had been raped as a young girl by a relative. She said that she had never told anyone, not her parents or her spouse. She said she couldn't believe she was telling me now. She said she had decided long ago to forget it, never speak of it, never even think of it. We talked then about this memory being held in the thigh muscles, never released or acknowledged. She decided to use the crabapple remedy to help her release this memory and its tension and to help her jettison the hidden feelings of guilt, shame, and "dirtiness." Following ten days of treatment with the flower remedy and one more session using the polarity balancing (electromagnetic pulses) and carnelian stone, the tension in Julie's thighs relaxed.

CASE 2

I met Maureen at a dream seminar. When she discovered that I worked with a variety of natural therapies, she began to tell me about a knee problem she had recently developed. She believed it to be the result of a significant weight gain she had put on in the past year, thought the extra weight was probably straining her knee in some way. About a week later, Maureen called and made an appointment for a polarity therapy session. Maureen was forty-eight years old, divorced and very excited about returning to school. She had just begun clases and believed this to be a very important step for her. She seemed a little "hyper" and agitated when she arrived for her session; I attributed this to her recent new challenges and demands in school. About half way through the session, she became increasingly restless and finally suggested that we take a short break while she collected herself and used the bathroom. I was feeling that the session was perhaps not going to be as productive as it could be because of the restlessness, interruptions and lack of centeredness.

We proceeded with the remaining part of her body-work and I moved on to balance and assess the chakra centers. I found both the sacral and throat chakras to be disturbed, the throat center being the more imbalanced of the two. Her knee problem I had suspected might be a side-effect of a polarity disturbance of the triple warmer meridian; since this meridian networks to the sacral center, the imbalance there seemed justifiable. But since the throat center was the more imbalanced of the two, I anointed the throat reflex points with sassafras oil and placed a piece of obsidian (stone which resonates the throat chakra) in her left hand. I then placed the crystals against the soles of her feet to amplify the obsidian energy, and quietly awaited the balancing of the foot pulses. Maureen seemed to relax markedly during this part of the session. After holding the crystals in place for about four minutes, she remarked that the stone she was holding (the obsidian) felt very hot and tingly. In another minute or so the foot pulses balanced, we finished the session and I helped her up from the table.

She was sitting in one of my office chairs, putting on her shoes, when she suddenly broke into wracking sobs. Her emotional expression was so extreme and intense that at first I was a little alarmed. I thought she was going to collapse. Her whole body was shaking, shuddering with her sobs and the tears were streaming down her cheeks. She began to tell me about a series of losses she had experienced, one after another, about eighteen months ago. The string of disasters she recounted included the separate accidental deaths of both her sons and the destruction of her home. She said she had not been able to mourn or even cry at either of the funerals, that she'd been taught as a girl that tears were a waste of time, "like closing the barn door after the cows got out," she said. She realized that she had suppressed her grief, never completed the grieving process, and was wondering aloud if perhaps her weight gain was symbolic of her unshed tears, a burden of grief that she was accumulating and carrying around with her. Maureen wept almost continuously for the next twelve hours. She continued to be very emotionally sensitive for more than a week, sometimes breaking into tears. Though this was a little unnerving to her, she understood the process of her own release and healing, and this knowledge helped her make it through this period. We continued to see each other for several months following our initial session. She began to make progress losing the extra weight, and the knee problem disappeared almost immediately. Through the first two weeks following her initial treatment, Maureen used both hyssop and hawthorn flower remedies to assist her in releasing and experiencing her grief. Her emotions seemed to stabilize after the third week.

It had been my observation in the past, in other sessions with other clients, that periods of grief, shock, or trauma often disturbed the sacral chakra and the triple warmer meridian. In one other case of unexpressed grief both the sacral and the throat centers had been disturbed. This leads me to speculate that possibly the sacral center is affected by *expressed* grief, while the throat center seems to be affected by *unexpressed* grief.

CASE 3

Kay had been a student in several of my workshops. She was a social-worker, deeply dedicated to her work and interested in holistic healing. She was currently working with adolescent substance abusers and was eager to learn about any natural healing methods which might help her work with these children. Kay was in her late forties, trim, and physically active. She had experienced several other forms of bodywork, including Rolfing, and was curious about polarity and chakra balancing. She scheduled a short series of sessions "to see what would happen." During the course of our first session together, I noticed one of her hips was higher than the other, and the pelvis was slightly twisted. I have found that this postural picture often coincides with a disturbance of the circulation meridian. In assessing and balancing the chakra centers during the session, I found the sacral center imbalanced; the center to and from which the circulation meridian networks. I anointed the skull base with clove oil and placed the carnelian in her left hand for polarity intake, holding the crystals against her feet to amplify the carnelian vibration. The bodywork and balancing session went quietly.

It is my habit to schedule a short time following the bodywork session when the client and I can sit down together and discuss the tensions located during the treatment and develop a program of exercise and therapy to correct these situations. After our session, we sat down to talk about these things. I told her about the pelvic misalignment and about how I often found this to be a problem with the circulation meridian. This meridian, I told her, is often disturbed during periods of sexual transition. I wondered (and asked her) if she was perhaps experiencing menopause. Her face fell as soon as I mentioned it. She told me that several years ago she had had a hysterectomy even though there was no clinical or pathological reason to do so. She said there had been a history of late pregnancies in her family. She felt that at this stage in her life she wanted to concentrate on her career and she did not want to be worried about or burdened by a pregnancy. Her fear of this possible pregnancy was so great, she said, that she went from one doctor to another until she found a doctor who would perform the surgery. Deep down inside, she said, she felt this was the coward's way out and the wrong thing to do. She almost cancelled the surgery at the last minute, but in the end, she went through with it. Kay went on to say that since that time (about three years) she had had very uneasy feelings about this decision and felt that she had secretly denied life to another being. She said she even investigated adopting a child to somehow "make up" for this decision. She felt that her current work was also a type of "penance." Kay and I worked together for several months, using flower remedies and bodywork to assist in releasing her past "mistake."

GLOSSARY

acupoint: electromagnetic centers located along bioenergy circuits (meridians) which function much like an electrical resistor to adjust the speed and force of energy traveling along the circuit. There are more than 500 acupoints commonly used to adjust body energies.

acupressure: the use of neuropressure massage on acupoint locations for the purpose of adjusting bioenergies; "fingertip acupuncture."

acute: situation of rapid onset, marked symptoms, and short duration or course.

adrenal gland: endocrine gland located above each kidney; its secretions markedly affect the nervous and cardiovascular systems, metabolic rate, temperature and smooth muscle action. It is the primary glandular responder in the "fight or flight" reaction and is esoterically associated with the sacral chakra.

alterative: a therapeutic agent which detoxifies body tissues by improving cellular nutrition and elimination; utilized primarily in blood poisoning and impurities, toxemia, pH imbalance and systemic toxicity.

antiseptic: a therapeutic agent which inhibits or destroys microbial and bacterial growth; employed in infectious and septic conditions.

antispasmodic: a therapeutic agent which relaxes muscle tissue by decreasing electrical excitability in nervous tissue; employed in muscular spasm, cramp, and pain due to muscular tension.

aromatherapy: the therapeutic application of scent and essential oils which acts primarily on the nervous system and emotional body.

aufu body: (Egyptian) the physical body; alchemically correspondent to the earth element.

autonomic nervous system (ANS): the portion of the nervous system which regulates involuntary body functions such as glandular response and smooth muscle contraction. Via the endocrine glands, the ANS generates a wide range of physical states including hunger sensation, metabolic rate, body temperature, blood pressure, pulse, and sensory acuity.

bonham corpuscles: small oval electromagnetic cells surrounding skin capillaries and blood vessels.

brow chakra: physiological and psychological developmental center correspondent with the pituitary gland. Esoterically identified with the evolution of leadership and group integration expression and the urge for power and control. The brow chakra represents the higher octave expression of the navel center forces of personal desire and emotion.

cardiac: pertaining to the heart; a therapeutic agent which tones heart muscle and regulates or normalizes heart rhythm.

catabolic: the destructive breakdown phase of metabolism, converting complex substances into simple ones usually for the purposes of elimination or energy release; a therapeutic agent which stimulates the breakdown-excretion phase of metabolism, used primarily in situations of encysted material, abscess or obesity.

central meridian: one of the two main bioenergy circuits, located on the front of the body between the pubis and lower lip; the yin-negative electromagnetic storage circuit.

chakra: Sanskrit word for "wheel"; a bioenergy vortex and its glandular counterpart, esoterically identified as a multilevel human developmental center, integrating physical, psychological and spiritual evolution.

chromotherapy: the therapeutic use of color and of spectrum refraction in gems.

chronic: situation of slow, progressive development and long continuance or duration.

crown chakra: physiological and psychological developmental center correspondent with the pineal gland. Esoterically identified as the center for evolution of the intuitive capacity, essence experience and self-actualization. The crown chakra represents the higher octave expression of the solar plexus forces of personal mind, intelligence, and communication.

demulcent: a therapeutic agent which acts as an anti-inflammatory, soothing, softening or shielding membranes; employed in inflammation, abrasion, irritation, i.e., wounds, burns.

diaphoretic: a therapeutic agent which decreases body temperature by increasing heat loss through the skin; employed primarily in fever.

digestive-stomachic: a therapeutic agent which regulates or normalizes gastric enzymes and secretions; primarily utilized in gastric upset due to acid imbalance such as heartburn, gastritis, dyspepsia.

diuretic: a therapeutic agent which stimulates the production and excretion of urine; used primarily in water retention.

electromagnetic field: the force field surrounding and emanating from moving electric charges. The field has both magnetic and electric properties and these energies can be defined and measured.

emmenagogue: a therapeutic agent which promotes or assists the menstrual flow.

endocrine glands: ductless glands which produce internal secretions (hormones) which are discharged directly into the blood or lymph and circulated to all parts of the body. The endocrine glands include the pineal, pituitary, thyroid, gonads, adrenals, and parathyroids. Hormone secretions may specifically effect organs or tissues, or may exhibit general effects on the entire body. Included among the processes affected by hormones are metabolic rate, physical growth and development, reproductive system maturity and sexual development, development of personality and higher nervous functions, and the ability to cope with stress and disease.

expectorant: a therapeutic agent which promotes the expulsion of mucous from the respiratory tract.

fontanelle: French for "little fountain"; the unossified space or "soft spot" between cranial bones.

gonads: male and female sex glands (ovaries and testes) which form cells for human reproduction and secrete hormones which regulate the reproductive cycle. Esoterically associated with the navel chakra.

governor meridian: one of two main bioenergy storage circuits, located on the back of the body between the tailbone and the top of the lip; the yang-positive electromagnetic storage circuit.

haidit body: (Egyptian) the dream or emotional body associated with the unconscious mind; alchemically correspondent with the water element.

heart chakra: physiological and psychological developmental center correspondent with the thymus gland. Esoterically identified as the center for the evolution of idealism, expansion of self, and world-view. It is a conversion center for transferring energies of the lower octave chakras to the three higher chakras.

homeopathy: from Greek "homoios" (similar) and "pathos" (suffering). A school of medicine based on the theory that substances which elicit particular reactions or symptoms in a healthy person when given in a material or toxic dose can be utilized to alleviate similar conditions when given in minute micro-dosages.

ion: a sub-atomic particle containing an electrical charge.

ka body: (Egyptian) mental or intellectual body, the body of the conscious mind; alchemically correspondent to the element air.

khu body: (Egyptian) the body of the collective consciousness, alchemically correspondent to the element fire.

lymphatic: pertaining to the lymph system; a therapeutic agent which stimulates and regulates the lymphatic glandular function, promoting lymphocyte production and action, and supporting or reinforcing the immune response; used primarily to rebuild an impaired immune system, regulate allergic response and combat internal infection.

mantra: Sanskrit word meaning "prayer"; vibrational syllables (or syllable combinations) which integrate forces and forms.

meridian: bioenergy circuits which convey electromagnetic energy throughout the body. Although the meridians form a continuous circuit, for the purpose of study and therapy they are usually divided into fourteen principle circuits based on polarity value, and the organs and tissues supplied.

mudra: Sanskrit meaning "sign"; the gestural correlate of mantra. A mudra is a hand movement, or posture, which produces a vibrational resonance, and is both invocative and evocative, integrating forces and forms.

muscle insertion: the tendon end of a muscle which attaches to the movable bone.

muscle origin: the tendon end of a muscle which attaches to the most stationary bone.

myotherapy: muscle treatment; massage therapy.

navel chakra: physiological and psychological developmental center correspondent with the gonad glands. Esoterically identified as the center for evolution of the personal desire and emotion force, the will to have, to love, and the urge for security and belonging.

nephritic: a therapeutic agent which strengthens and supports the urinary tract organs and function.

nervine: a therapeutic agent which has mild tranquilizing and pain-relieving properties; used in minor pain, nervous tension, and agitation.

pancreas: functions both as an endocrine and exocrine gland; secreting enzymes and hormones which regulate glucose (sugar) metabolism and the blood sugar level. Esoterically associated with the solar plexus chakra.

piezoelectricity: the electrical pulse generated in pressurized crystals; used in radios, computers and timepieces.

pineal: endocrine gland situated in the third ventricle of the brain. There are three hormone-like substances secreted by the pineal gland, but their functions are not fully understood. Esoterically, the pineal gland is identified with the intuitive mind and faculties and the evolution of transcendent states of consciousness and self-actualization.

pituitary gland: endocrine gland located in the brain attached to the hypothalamus (just behind the root of the nose). It is often referred to as the "master gland" because of the wide range of bodily activities which it coordinates by regulating the function of other glands. Esoterically associated with the brow chakra.

polarity: the separation of positive and negative electrically charged particles, resulting in concentration or alignment of forces about opposing positions or "poles."

polarity therapy: a form of treatment in which the healer utilizes his or her own body to create a temporary circuit for the purpose of readjusting and realigning the electromagnetic energies in the recipient's body. The healer uses "points" or "poles" on the recipient's body to modulate and transfer energies.

prone: lying horizontal with the face downward; lying on the stomach.

radiesthesia: the use of a pendulum or dowsing device to detect fluctuations in an electromagnetic field.

resistor: an element in an electrical circuit which functions to inhibit or retard energy moving along the circuit; used to adjust and regulate energy flow.

sacral chakra: physiological and psychological developmental center correspondent with the adrenal glands. Esoterically identified as the center for evolution of the will to identity and autonomy and the urge for action and survival.

sahu body: (Egyptian) the causal body linking the physical body and its subtler counterparts with the divine level of being; alchemically correspondent to the "lapis" or philosopher's stone; the essential, authentic self.

sheng cycle: the "creation" cycle of bioenergy circuits which describes the dynamic relationship between meridians, helping the therapist to assess and realign meridian energies.

shiatsu: from Japanese "shi" meaning finger and "atsu" meaning pressure; pressure point therapy used to adjust meridian energies.

solar plexus chakra: physiological and psychological developmental center correspondent with the spleen and pancreas. Esoterically identified as the center for evolution of personal mind, the will to know and learn, and the urge to communicate.

spleen: the largest mass of lymphatic tissues in the body, located in the abdominal cavity just behind and below the stomach. In addition to filtering bacteria and antigens from the blood and producing lymphocytes to combat infection and establish immunity, the spleen also removes and disposes of worn out red blood cells and platelets, and stores and releases blood in the event of hemorrhage. Esoterically associated with the solar plexus chakra.

stimulant: a therapeutic agent which increases and normalizes blood circulation; used primarily to correct congestion and impaired circulation.

subtle body: a non-phenomenal or non-physical vehicle of human development and evolution; *see*, Ka, Khu and Haidit.

supine: lying on the back with the face upwards.

throat chakra: physiological and psychological developmental center correspondent with the thyroid gland. Esoterically identified as the center for evolution of creative focus, self-discipline, initiative and responsibility.

thymus gland: lymphatic tissue located in the upper chest just behind and above the heart. During childhood the thymus produces T-Cells and establishes the body's immune response. It is usually found atrophied and non-functional by early adulthood. Esoterically associated with the heart chakra.

thyroid gland: endocrine gland found in the neck. The thyroid's hormone secretions regulate the metabolic rate and calcium level in the blood. Esoterically associated with the throat chakra.

transducer: from Latin, "to lead across"; a substance or device which converts input energy of one form into output energy of another.

vibrational therapy: the therapeutic application of forms or substances (essential oil, gems, polarity balancing, color, homeopathic remedy) which act primarily by affecting or altering electromagnetic wave patterns. Vibrational therapies represent chemical potencies in higher vibrational octaves.

yantra: a visual, symbolic representation of a resonant, vibrational reality used to evoke or invoke particular states for healing or meditation.

yang: oriental term used to designate the positive polarity quality; associated with the sun and masculine forms, the left brain and right side of the body, and with states of movement, action, expansion, extroversion, and involvement.

yang meridians: bioenergy circuits which convey positive polarity energy throughout the body. The yang meridians include the stomach, urinary bladder, large and small intestine, gall bladder, triple warmer, and the main yang storage circuit—the governor meridian.

yin: oriental term used to designate negative polarity quality; associated with the moon and feminine forms of energy, with the right brain and left side of the body, and with states of receptivity, repose, introversion, contraction, and conservation.

yin meridians: bioenergy circuits which convey negative polarity energy throughout the body. The yin meridians include the heart, lung, liver, spleen, kidney, circulation, and the main yin storage circuit—the central meridian.

BIBLIOGRAPHY

Airola, Paavo. *How to Get Well*. Phoenix, AZ: Health Plus Publishers, 1974.

Anderson, Mary. *Color Healing*. York Beach, ME: Samuel Weiser, 1978; and Wellingborough, England: Thorsons Publishing Group, 1978.

Arroyo, Stephen. *Astrology, Psychology and the Four Elements*. Sebastopol, CA: CRCS, 1975.

Bach, Dr. Edward. *The Bach Flower Remedies*. New Canaan, CT: Keats Publishing, 1975.

———. *Heal Thyself*. Saffron Walden, England: C. W. Daniel, 1975.

Bailey, Alice. *Treatise on White Magic*. New York: Lucis Publishing, 1977.

Baumal, B. J. *Dictionary of Gesture*. Metuchen, NJ: Scarecrow Press, 1975.

Boericke, M. D., William. *Materia Medica With Repertory*. New Delhi, India: Jain, 1976.

Chancellor, Philip. *Handbook of the Bach Flower Remedies*. Saffron Walden, England: C. W. Daniel, 1974.

Colton, Anna Ree. *Watch Your Dreams*. Glendale, CA: Arc Publishing, 1977.

Cousins, Norman. *Anatomy of An Illness as Perceived by the Patient*. Los Angeles: Cancer House, 1979.

Critchley, M. *Silent Language*: London: Butterworth, 1975.

Cummings, Stephen and Dana Ullman. *Everybody's Guide to Homeopathic Medicines*. Los Angeles: Jeremy Tarcher, 1984.

Dass, Ram. *The Seed*. Albuquerque: Lama Foundation, 1974.

Diamond, M. D., John. *Your Body Doesn't Lie*. New York: Warner Books, 1979.

Ekman, P. and Frieson, W. V. *Unmasking the Face*. Englewood, NJ: Prentice-Hall, 1975.

Evans, J. A. *Magical Jewels of the Middle Ages and Renaissance*. New York: Dover, 1979.

Feldenkrais, Moshe. *Awareness through Movement*. New York: Harper & Row, 1972.

Glick, J. and J. Larusso. *Healing Stoned: The Therapeutic Use of Gems & Minerals*. Albuquerque, NM: Brotherhood of Life, 1979.

Gurudas. *Flower Essences*. Albuquerque, NM: Brotherhood of Life, 1983.

Harding, M. E. *Psychic Energy: Its Source & Transformation*. Princeton, NJ: Princeton University Press, 1973.

Jones, T. W. Hynes. *Dictionary of the Bach Flower Remedies*. C. W. Daniel, Saffron Walden, England: 1977.

Jung, Carl G. *The Collected Works*. Tr. by R. F. C. Hull. Princeton, NJ: Princeton University Press, 1953.

Kapit, W. and L. Elson. *The Anatomy Coloring Book*. New York: Harper & Row, 1977.

Karlfried, Graf von Durkheim. *Daily Life as Spiritual Exercise*. London: Unwin & Hyman, 1971.

Kent, M. D., James. *Repertory Materia Medica*. Chicago: Ehrhard & Karl, 1957.

Kreiger, Delores. *Therapeutic Touch*. Englewood, NJ: Prentice-Hall, 1979.

Kumz, George. *Curious Lore of Precious Stones*. New York: Dover, 1971.

Lautie, R. and Andre Passebecq, M.D. *Aromatherapy*. Aylesbury, England, 1979; now out of print.

Leadbeater, C. W. *The Chakras*. Wheaton, IL: Theosophical Publishing, 1972.

Luscher, Dr. Max. *The Luscher Color Test*. New York: Washington Square Press, 1971.

Maslow, Abraham. "Self Actualization & Beyond" in *Challenges in Humanistic Psychology*. New York: McGraw-Hill, 1967.

Masters, Robert. "The Way of the Five Bodies" in *Aquarian Changes*, Vol. 5 No. 2. April, 1983.

Medicines for the New Age. Virginia Beach, VA: Heritage, 1977.

Mermet, Abbe. *Principles and Practices of Radiesthesia*. Shaftesbury, England: Element Books, 1987.

Rolf, Ida. *Rolfing: The Integration of Human Structures*. New York: Harper & Row, 1978.

Samuels, Michael and Nancy. *Seeing With the Mind's Eye*. New York: Random House, 1975.

Schwaller de Lubicz, Isha. *Her-Bak: The Living Face of Ancient Egypt*. Rochester, VT: Inner Traditions, 1978.

______. *Her-Bak: Egyptian Initiate*. Rochester, VT: Inner Traditions, 1978.

______. *Opening of the Way*. Rochester, VT: Inner Traditions, 1978.

Schwaller de Lubicz, R. A. *The Temple in Man*. Rochester, VT: Inner Traditions, 1979.

Sontag, Susan. *Illness as Metaphor*. New York: Vintage Press, 1979.

Sourindro, M. Tagore. *Yantra*. New York: AMS Press, 1976.

Stone, Randolph. *Polarity Therapy, Wireless Anatomy of Man*. Sebastopol, CA: CRCS, 1986.

Tappan, F. *Healing Massage Techniques*. Englewood, NJ: Prentice-Hall, 1980.

Thie, John. *Touch for Health*. Marina del Rey, CA: DeVorss, 1979.

Thompson, William. *The Time Falling Bodies Take to Light*. New York: St. Martin's Press, 1981.

Tisserand, Robert. *Aromatherapy*. Rochester, VT: Inner Traditions, 1977.

Ulyldert, M. *The Magic of Precious Stones*. Wellingborough, England: Thorsons Publishing Group, 1979.

Wheeler, F. J. *The Bach Remedies Repertory*. Saffron Walden, England: C. W. Daniel, 1974.

Whitmont, Edward. *Psyche & Substance: Essays on Homeopathy in the Light of Jungian Psychology*. Richmond, CA: North Atlantic Books, 1980.

Yellow Emperor's Classic of Internal Medicine. Tr. Ilza Veith. Berkeley, CA: University of California Press, 1966.

SUGGESTED READING

Besant, Annie. *Man & His Bodies*. Wheaton, IL: Theosophical Publishing House, 1967.

Hall, Manly P. *Occult Anatomy of Man*. Los Angeles: Philosophical Research Society, 1957.

______. *The Secret Teachings*. Los Angeles: Philosophical Research Society, 1967.

Heindel, Max. *Rosicrucian Cosmo-Conception*. Oceanside, CA: Rosicrucian Fellowship, 1954.

______. *The Vital Body*. Oceanside, CA: Rosicrucian Fellowship, 1957.

______. *The Ductless Glands*. Oceanside, CA: Rosicrucian Fellowship, 1972.

Jung, Carl G. *The Undiscovered Self*. New York: Mentor Books, 1958.

Kreiger, Delores. *Therapeutic Touch*. Englewood, NJ: Prentice-Hall, 1979.

Maslow, Abraham. *Motivation & Personality*. New York: Harper & Row, 1954.

Motoyama, Hiroshi. *Theories of the Chakras: Bridge to Higher Consciousness*. Wheaton, IL: Theosophical Publishing House, 1981.

Powell, A. E. *Mental Body*. Wheaton, IL: Theosophical Publishing House, 1975.

______. *Astral Body*. Wheaton, IL: Theosophical Publishing House, 1978.

______. *Causal Body*. Wheaton, IL: Theosophical Publishing House, 1972.

______. *Etheric Body*. Wheaton, IL: Theosophical Publishing House, 1979.

RESOURCES FOR REMEDIES AND INFORMATION

Bach Flower Remedies

The Dr. Edward Bach Centre
Mount Vernon
Sotwell, Wallingford
Oxon OX10 0PZ
England
Phone: +44-1491 834678
Fax: +44-1491 825022
e-mail: bachcentre.com

Institut für Bach-Blütentherapie
Forschung und Lehre
Mechthild Scheffer
Lippmannstrasse 53
D-22769 Hamburg
Germany
Phone: +49-40-43 25 77 10
Fax: +49-40-43 52 53
e-mail: info@bach-bluetentherapie.de

Flower Essences

The Flower Essence Services
P. O. Box 1769
Nevada City, CA 95959
Phone: (800)548-0075
Fax: (530)265-6467
Web: www.floweressence.com

Homeopathic Remedies

The following companies in the United States carry remedies in both tablet and liquid form, as well as books and information on the subject of homeopathy:

Homeopathic Educational Services
2124 Kittredge Street
Berkeley, CA 94704
Phone: (510)649-0294
Fax: (510)649-1955
Web: www.homeopathic.com
(They also carry books and information on the Bach Flower Remedies.)

Standard Homeopathic Company
P. O. Box 61067
Los Angeles, CA 90061
Phone: (800)624-9659
Fax: (310)516-8579

International Resources for Homeopathic Remedies. Contact for information and current prices.

Ainsworth Homeopathic Pharmacy
36 New Cavendish Street
London W1M 7LH
England
Phone: +44-171 935 5330
Fax: +44-171 486 4313

Martin and Pleasance Wholesale
123 Dover Street
Richmond, Victoria
3121
Australia
Phone: +61-3-9427 7422
Fax: +61-3-9428 8431
e-mail: jeremyct@ozemail.com.au

Essential Oils

Penn Herb Company
10601 Decatur Road
Philadelphia, PA 19154
Phone: (800)523-9971
Fax: (215)632-7945
e-mail: orders@pennherb.com
Web: www.pennherb.com

INDEX